Comments from early reviewers...

"There are lots of books on the single life, but this one is special. It's packed with fresh insights you won't find anywhere else. Lewis' advice, particularly on communicating with men and being choosy in a healthy way, is solid gold."

—Florence Isaacs, author of *Toxic Friends/True Friends: How Your Friends Can Make or Break Your Health, Happiness, Family, and Career* (Morrow)

"At last there is a popular book available that portrays single women as authentic individuals who can have rich and fulfilling lives. Without romancing the single state, Dr. Lewis addresses the challenges and opportunities it affords single women. Peppered with humor and wisdom, this book provides a unique and empowering view of single women while at the same time supplying well needed suggestions and a heavy dose of support and comfort."

—Natalie Schwartzberg, author of *Single in a Married World: A Life Cycle Framework for Working with the Unmarried Adult*

"A thoughtful look at women's lives today. Savvy and encouraging, like having a good friend in your corner as you face life's challenges. A good read for any man who cares about the women in his life as well."

—Sam Osherson, PhD, author of *Wrestling With Love: How Men Struggle with Intimacy*

"A deceptively easy read, *With or Without a Man* provides a framework for understanding why being single in our culture can be so difficult. Lewis, an always single family therapist, has written a thorough and authoritative book that can allow single women to stop blaming themselves for being single and to start taking charge of their lives. She helps readers name the unspoken and fashion strategies that can lead to a satisfying life with or without a man. This book is a must read!"

—Beth M. Erickson, author of *Longing for Dad: Father Loss and Its Impact* and *Helping Men Change: The Role of the Female Therapist*

"*With or Without a Man* is a fresh and sparkling treatment of a subject treated so dreadfully in other books. Karen Gail Lewis understands single women in all their diversity, and offers astute and balanced insights about men as well. Ultimately, this is a book of wisdom about living a healthy life, no matter what your marital situation or marital prospects. Bravo, Karen!"

—William J. Doherty, author of *The International Family* and *Take Back Your Kids: Confident Parenting in Turbulent Times*

"If it weren't for wanting to be with a man, the single life can be quite satisfying." Psychotherapist Lewis hits the nail on the head in her seminal handbook for heterosexual women who are postponing living full, "adult lives" because they're biding their time in what they hope is the transitional stage of being single. All women, whether married or single, she asserts, have the same basic needs for intimacy, a healthy self-image and sexual expression; without a man, a single woman must work more diligently to fulfill each of these fundamental needs. To help women do so, Lewis offers nine worthy "tasks" ("being grounded," "making a decision about children," etc.), followed by opportunities for reflection and self assessment—a well-thought-out road map for women to travel beyond feeling overwhelmed by value judgments (theirs and everyone else's) about why they're not married. She encourages women in their mid-30s to their late-60s to recognize "this distinction: You have no control over when an appropriate man will fit in your life, but you do have control over making the life that you have a good one—for however long you have it." Well written, motivational and practical, Lewis's guide offers single women fresh and detailed advice for creating a happy, meaningful life. Like the 1995 bestselling *Flying Solo*, Lewis's book provides single women with a bracing perspective—and an action plan. With its broad appeal, this title is well suited for reading groups.

—(October, 23, 2000 issue of *Publisher's Weekly* Forecasts)

"This is a gold mine for single women. It covers all the issues that need to be considered, offering sensitive insight and practical suggestions while putting everything in the context of the vast changes in society's 'rules' for single women."

—Betty Carter, MSW, Director Emeritus, Family Institute of Westchester, New York.

With Or Without Man

Single Women Taking Control Of Their Lives

Richard –
your life needs to
be fulfilled –
with or without a
woman –
Karen

By Karen Gail Lewis

Published by Bull Publishing Company, Post Office Box 208, Palo Alto, California 94302-0208 (www.bullpub.com) in association with Lansing Hays Publishing LLC, 248 Prince George Street, Annapolis, Maryland 21401

Typeset in 10 pt. Sabon with ITC Kabel.
Printer: Malloy Printing
Interior design: Jeff Klavon
Cover: Lightbourne Design
Author photo: Sarah Greene, Greene Graphics, Milton,DE.
Managing and copy editor: Linda O'Doughda

04 03 02 01   5 4 3 2

Library of Congress Cataloging-in-Publication Data

Lewis,Karen Gail.
    With or without a man : taking control of your life as a single woman / by Karen Gail Lewis.
      p. cm.
    Includes bibliographical references and index.
    ISBN 0-923521-50-X
      1. Single women. I. Title.

  HQ800.2.L49 2000
  305.48'9652--dc21
                                                                            00-056434
  British Library Cataloguing-in-Publication Data

  A CIP record is available from the British Library

Printed in the United States of America
First Edition

Dedication

In memory of my father, who encouraged me to take the time to write this, and my uncle, who was a good role model of a single adult.

Table Of Contents

Preface

"What's wrong with me that I'm not married?" asks Patsy, a petite dark-haired, dark-eyed physician. Her sentence echoes inside my head, for I had heard the exact same words an hour before from Nancy, a tall, blonde legal assistant. So, on a Wednesday afternoon, in the middle of a therapy session, I make a decision. I have to write a book about single women.

Later that same Wednesday afternoon, in the middle of another session, I confirm my decision to write this book. A stocky, red-haired bank teller named Ruth has just comfortably remarked: "You know, being single is a fact of my life, along with lots of other facts. I would like to have a husband, and I would like to have fewer freckles. But you don't always get what you want in this world."

Single women come in all heights, hair colors, personalities, and professions, and they have a variety of feelings about being single. Therefore, I write this book for all the Patsys and Nancys who wonder what's wrong with them and for all the Ruths who are content being single but wouldn't mind being married.

The purpose of this book is *not* to argue for the single life or to help you stop being single. The purpose is to help you take control of your life—whatever it is at the moment. You are single now, so make it the best life you can, for however long you are there. If you become partnered or married, make that the best life, for however long you are there.

The Research Study

The information for this book comes from several sources. First, I draw from my more than 30 years of professional experience as a social worker, psychologist, and family therapist. I have heard so many of the same comments from women from different walks of life—white women and women of color, rich and poor—that I can no longer view their stories as isolated experiences. These stories reflect a sociological phenomenon about today's midlife single women.

I also draw from my own experience of being single. That has been for 56, 35, or 26 years, depending on whether you begin counting from birth, when I turned 21, or when I entered my 30s. I have also gathered information from my single friends.

To add to the discourse, I intended to interview six to eight women who were neither clients nor friends. I put a four-line announcement in *The Washington Post* asking Always Single and Single Again women between the ages of 30 and 65 to participate in a small group interview.

To my surprise, by 7:00 PM of the day the ad appeared, I had already heard from 40 women. By the end of the first week, more than 200 had called for more information. Clearly, women wanted a chance to talk about being single. I had to quickly redesign my research.

Based on that new design, the study reports on nine small group interviews with 45 Always Single and Single Again women. Each group interview lasted about three hours. It also includes responses to an extensive, 17-page questionnaire that I mailed to an additional 45 single women.

These two different formats allowed for more in-depth exploration of the issues, as well as an understanding of how women manage their public and private, their conscious and unconscious, views about being single.

The examples from my clients and the women in the study have been altered to protect their confidentiality. The names have been changed and the details and circumstances have been used to create composite stories that are not directly related to any one person.

Let Me Introduce Myself

As I present this material around the country, I'm faced with contradictory reactions. Many women resonate with the ideas and feel relieved hearing them. Some, though, accuse me of being a man-hater. That's not true. The accusations against me may be an excuse for not seriously examining these concepts.

These accusations, though, raise the question of who I am. So, let me tell you something about me. But what should I tell you?

- That I am an Always Single 56-year-old heterosexual woman with no children?

- That I am a loved and appreciated daughter and sister; have a very close relationship with my nieces and nephew; am a valued friend?

- That I recently lost my long-time companion, Indie, who was part Doberman and part German shepherd?

- That I am a social worker, psychologist, and family therapist with nine diplomas on my wall; the author of four books and many professional articles?

- That I have had several important love relationships in the past; have been without one for several years; have recently been in one and am uncertain where it will go?

Which of these facts qualifies me for writing this book? Do any of them make me more eligible or more suspect? Since I am single, will I write from an embittered position, or will I tout the advantages of being single? Am I too close to a subject that touches me personally? These are reasonable questions to ponder as you decide whether this is a book worth reading. The real question, though, is, Can I use my professional and personal experiences in ways that are helpful rather than distorting?

Acknowledgments

I owe a great debt to the women who participated in the study I conducted on single women; they shared their life stories and their private emotions. I also am indebted to the many women and men, single and married, I have had the privilege of working with over the past three decades. Finally, I am indebted to my single women friends who have more than willingly shared their stories and given me feedback on some of the chapters.

Several women gathered on Wednesday evenings during the cold autumn and winter months to discuss their thoughts and reactions to working drafts of the manuscript. I thank Pam Kane, Ann Prost, Jinny Spencer, and Wanda Stansbury for their camaraderie and for their suggestions, which I have tried to incorporate.

Enormous thanks to my publisher, Lansing Hays, who although a man and married, saw the importance of these ideas and made this book possible. Another enormous thank you to Linda O'Doughda for her perceptive and precise editing.

And, finally, unending gratitude to my mother and father, my brothers Doug and Steve, my sister-in-law Linda, my nieces Misha, Deborah, Ami, and Naomi, and my nephew Daniel for enriching my life—whether I was with or without a man.

Dr. Karen Gail Lewis is available for lectures for the general public and workshops and training presentations for mental health professionals.
She can be reached as follows:
Dr. Karen Gail Lewis
560 N Street, SW
Suite N505
Washington, DC 20024
301-585-5814

With Or Without A Man

Single Women Taking Control Of Their Lives

Introduction

If it weren't for wanting to be with a man, the single life can be quite satisfying. Research shows what single women already know: They can have a rich and fulfilling life without marriage. In fact, they often are more self-reliant and feel more centered than their married friends since they have had more space to devote to their self-development.

With or Without a Man starts with the premise that you know how to meet men and what to do on dates. It makes the assumption that you, like most women, are working on your personal growth—either through having read books, talked with friends, or been in therapy.

With or Without a Man is different from other self-help books in its explanation for why there are so many single women today: More women than men are pursuing their personal growth, so *more women than men are ready for a healthy relationship*. And, women only want to be with emotionally healthy men.

We live in a society that values marriage as the "norm." If that value judgment were removed, being married and being single would be two equally viable paths through adulthood. There would be no need for women to blame themselves for being single.

Life is full of ambiguities, and for single women, a major one is not knowing if you'll meet a suitable man for a long-term relationship or marriage.

If you are in love, at this point in your life you know that that is not enough. Being in love is wonderful: there's a deep sense of connection and mutual nurturing. But, loving a man who cannot make a commitment to you, or who blocks your personal or professional growth, or who is not emotionally available, or who is emotionally or physically abusive is neither wonderful nor enough.

The reality is that whether or not a woman has a relationship with a man, she may feel something is missing if she isn't meeting her needs in the other areas of her life, separate from that relationship. These needs include a connection with close friends and a nurturance that comes from being involved in meaningful work or an avocation.

Since love is not static—there are romantic highs, times of being bored and unappreciated, unnerving arguments, the quiet depth of affection—you need a life that is rewarding, especially during the low points in a relationship, or if that relationship ends.

As a single woman, you have no control over meeting an emotionally available man, but you do have control over including intimacy and internal fulfillment in your life.

This book describes nine tasks to help you do this.

Who Is This Book For?

With or Without a Man speaks to heterosexual Always Single and Single Again women. An Always Single woman is one who has never been married, regardless of whether she is or has been in a long-term relationship. A Single Again woman is one who has returned to being single, either through divorce or her husband's death.

This book also speaks to women who may or may not want to be (re)married but who do want to be with a loving male. It speaks to women who are not dating because they are not meeting a man worth their time; to women who are dating but have no commitment from a man for an exclusive relationship; to women in a committed relationship. It speaks to women of all colors. While many issues about being single are related to one's ethnicity or race, my study suggests that living in America neutralizes most of the differences.

With or Without a Man specifically speaks to women in their mid-30s to late-60s. This time span is chosen because the issues are different for younger and older women. Today, women in their 20s claim they do not feel pressured to be married. They like having the time to pursue their career and explore meeting men and learn more about themselves in relationships. Once they turn 30, though, it's as if a timer starts. By their mid-30s, women more realistically grapple with the possibility of their never marrying.

Nevertheless, women in their 20s may find the information here helpful as a preventive guide for avoiding self-blame and enhancing their life in case they do not marry by their mid-30s.

The Structure Of The Book

With or Without a Man has three sections. Chapters 1 through 3 offer an understanding of our societal bias toward marriage and how that can affect a woman's feelings about herself as a single.

Chapters 4 through 12 describe nine tasks for living a satisfying single life—ignoring the societal bias. Weaving through each of these nine tasks is the basic human need for a deep connection with others. This comes from loving and being loved, neither of which is limited to romantic love alone.

The second basic need interwoven in each of the nine tasks is nurturing—nurturing yourself, nurturing others, and letting others nurture you. Without all three forms of nurturing, you may feel emotionally depleted, attributing that feeling to your not having a partner.

These nine tasks provide a structure for assessing whether or not you are getting the nourishing connections you need for a satisfying single life—with or without a man. The tasks can be used as a periodic checkup to see how well you are doing as an adult single.

Another way to use the tasks is to see where you experience the most pain in your life and then read the chapter that corresponds to that pain. You may well find clues for the causes and the cure.

A third way to use the tasks, especially on days when you're feeling blue, is to focus on all that you have accomplished, reminding yourself of the strength you possess in being an adult single in a world that values married couples.

A Self-Assessment checklist is included at the end of each task chapter. It is a fluid scale, changing as your week and your life change. When you are depressed or dissatisfied with your life, or aching for a man, check each section to see if you have let slip some of the ways to stay connected, to get nurtured. Look to see if that part of your life needs more nurturing or a deeper connection. This won't remove your ache to be touched and held, to be loved by and to love a man, but it will help you take control of having a satisfying single life until that happens—and beyond.

The three chapters that conclude the book (13–15) focus on teaching a man how to have a good relationship; describing therapy for single women; and calling for a Cultural Revolution, with suggestions for constructively mobilizing your anger at men and confronting—within yourself and within society—messages that blame you for being single.

Some women are better able than others to navigate the obstacles in our culture and free themselves from the societal messages described in the first three chapters. Therefore, they may find this material unnecessary. Feel free to skip these chapters and start with the task chapters, which affect all single women. Pick and choose the order of the tasks you want to read.

Getting Ready To Start

Shire Hite, in *Good Guys, Bad Guys* (Pandora Press, 1991), complains about self-help books for women.

> There is a certain insulting quality to many of the books that have appeared on women and relationships. They speak to women almost as if we were adolescents in waiting, "desperate for a man" or "desperate" for any new "instruction manual" on our "emotional dysfunction" (or "masochism"!) and ways to "fix ourselves" (p. 21).

I concur. It's insulting to teach people something they have been doing for years. Always Singles and long-time Single Agains do not need instructions. What they do need is a clearer understanding of the complexity of their feelings about being single, about the cause of their self-blame; they may need a description of life tasks, whether they are living with or without a man. They certainly need to hear there is not one blueprint for all single women.

With or Without a Man is not meant as a comparison between being single and being married. Where there are similarities, that only confirms the joys and struggles of all women. It is not meant as a comparison of issues between women and men. It simply focuses on the issues specifically for single women.

Throughout the pages, you will find a number of stereotypes and generalizations intended to facilitate the exploration of a concept. If you find them unhelpful, ignore them.

While everyone will read the same words, you may each read a different book, because you each bring your own life experience. You may recognize yourself on some pages and not on others. Where you don't, consider yourself fortunate, for you have been spared some issues that other women haven't.

Hopefully, some of the ideas will strike a resonating cord, confirm your own values, validate your confusion, help you challenge the internalized messages, and reeducate yourself and your loved ones.

An Up-Close And
Personal Look
At Today's Single Woman

It's a glorious Sunday morning. You can almost feel the buds pushing up through the ground. I wonder how many women will forgo this beautiful spring day to attend the meeting. Eight had signed up, but three canceled, deciding it was too upsetting to talk about being single. So, five women are expected.

It's 9:45 AM. I look around the room. What more do I need to do in the remaining 15 minutes? The chairs have been set in a circle; the video recorder is in place, and the mike has been tested. In the center of the room the small table is loaded with a jug of cider, a plate of pastries, glasses, plates, napkins.

There's a knock on the door. Someone always has to bear the awkwardness of being the first to arrive, but only for a short while, for by 10:15, all five women are seated and ready to go.

I commend the women for coming out on such a lovely day and sharing their insights with me. They can expect open-ended questions. I suggest that each one briefly introduce herself in terms of being a midlife single woman.

One Study Group

A short stocky woman with laughing eyes, dressed in black pants and top, offers to go first. "I'm Alysha. I'm 57 years young and getting better all the time. I was married for 17 years before I got sick of my husband taking me for granted, for putting me and the children second to his work, his drinking, his golf. I joke about it now, but divorcing him was really hard back then when there was no support for single mothers. But I managed; I'm a survivor. I have four grown kids, and three grandchildren. I've been single now for about 19 years.

"Since the kids have grown up, I've dated off and on, but frankly, I haven't met any men worth the trouble. I'd rather be lonely and unhappy by myself than lonely and unhappy with a man. Men just don't know how to talk to or be with women. [The other four women vigorously nod in agreement.] I'm not interested in dating now and certainly not in getting married again. I like my life—my work, my grandkids, my friends. I'm busy now thinking about my retirement. My latest idea is joining a circus as a clown!"

Alysha has a way of talking that puts the group at ease. The sense of relaxation in the room is almost palpable.

The woman sitting to her right, tall and thin, presents a sharp contrast in her bright red-and-purple pantsuit. "My name is Margaret, and next week I'll be 44." Several women simultaneously break into "Happy Birthday." The group has clearly warmed up.

Margaret thanks them and teases that they should take their show on the road. Then, in a more serious voice, she continues.

"I've never been married. I don't know if I ever want to marry, but I would love to meet someone I want to be with for life. I don't care if we live together. But that's not even an issue now because I haven't met a decent man for far too long. I'm mostly okay with that because, like you, Alysha, I have a really good life. I have my moments, though, when I just long for a man."

"I know what you mean about not meeting any decent men," says the woman next to Margaret. "I'm Doris. I had a short marriage when I was in my 20s. We were too young, and we both agreed it was a mistake. Then, eight years ago, I remarried. I thought we were so much in love, but he never wanted to make love with me. I kept wondering what was wrong with me and did everything I could to make myself more sexually attractive to him. But then I discovered he had been having a series of affairs since almost the first month after our wedding. I was devastated. It took me several years to get over feeling as if I were the most undesirable woman in the world. [Heads again nod, this time in empathy.]

"Unlike you two," Doris looks at Alysha and Margaret, "I put a lot of effort into trying to meet men but haven't found anyone that I can trust and who excites me. I need both. My friends (and my mother) think it's because I'm bitter at men. It's not true, though. I really do want to meet another man. I'm 41 and I still want children, so I feel a huge pressure to meet someone." Then Doris turns to her right, smiling as if to say, "Your turn."

Looking around the group, Bunny gives her name and says, "I may be the youngest one here. I'm 36. I've never been married. I was living with a man for four years, but we broke up a few years ago. I always knew it wasn't a good relationship. I don't know why I stayed. Maybe I was afraid to be alone. Marty wasn't mean or anything, but he didn't have any direction, and he clearly wasn't interested in marriage. Finally, he left. I wasn't devastated like you, Doris, but it was awful. I guess I just didn't want to go back out to the single world.

"Since then, I've dated a lot of men—lots—but none for more than a few months. I can understand the pressure you feel, Doris. I see the big 4-0 looming in my future, and I get scared I will be too old to be a mother. Besides that, I just want to be married." It wasn't a whine, but a clear, deep-felt wish. The room is quiet while Bunny and Doris exchange a silent moment together.

Breaking the silence, the last woman in the group jokes, "I guess I'll go next. You're the youngest, Bunny, and I'm the only widow. I'm Rita, and my husband died about 14 years ago. We'd been married for 12 years. I was in my mid-30s. A couple of years later, when my daughter was beginning to date, she wanted me to start going out again and teased me about double-dating! It was hard getting back out into the single world. I hated it.

"Since then, though, I've dated a few men. They've been okay, but none I would want to spend my life with. You have to be able to talk with a guy and feel he cares about what you have to say. There's obviously something wrong with me that I'm not meeting the right guy. My mother thinks I'm not over Larry, but I know it's not that. We had a decent marriage, but I have no assurance we wouldn't have gotten divorced if he had lived. No, it's not that. Maybe I'm just too fussy or too choosy."

The women break into an energetic discussion about "what's wrong with men." They comment about men's lack of sensitivity, their fear of commitment, their running away from intimacy. They tell jokes about men's inability to share their emotions with women.

"You ought to do a study about midlife single men," suggests Doris.

"Yeah, and I'd like to be a fly on the wall for it!" Bunny jests amidst the laughter.

Alysha, catching her breath, adds, "Can you imagine what they'd be talking about here? Sports, the stock market, the newest Microsoft programs. They'd say they try to get intimate with a woman by talking about these important topics, but all the women want to talk about is feelings!"

The bantering continues for a bit. As the energy begins to wane, I refocus the group by asking, "Why did you decide to participate in this study on midlife single women?" Their responses fall into two categories: they wanted to hear the experiences of other single women, and they want to help researchers understand what it's like being single.

Bunny giggles, "They need to hear what it's really like for us, not that glitzy stuff that gets portrayed on the TV and in the movies."

I then ask, "What's the best and worst thing about being single?"

I had barely finished my question when Doris spells out "R-e-l-i-e-f!" When the laughter subsides, she continues. "Not having to put up with a lot of jerks. I have freedom to walk away. I listen to my sisters complain about their marriages, and when I hang up the phone, I say, 'Thank goodness I don't have to deal with that stuff.'"

Bunny can barely wait until Doris finishes. "It's your independence. You can come and go, do what you want. Also, you don't have to clean up after a man." Although using the second person impersonal, she is clearly speaking for herself. "The drawback, though, is if you want to go someplace, there's no one to do it with."

"That's not an issue for me," says Margaret. "I have enough friends so that I can call someone and say let's go somewhere." She stops and repeats the question. "What's the best thing about being single? Having the freedom to work on me—who I am, where I'm going in my life. I can pay attention to my personal growth without having to deal with a husband and marriage problems. I also like not having to adjust my life, my schedule, especially my daily routine for a man. Let's see, the hardest part? Not having someone in your corner, someone who thinks you're great. Oh, yes, and sex. Not having a partner is really a problem; it puts pressure on you."

Alysha's eyes sparkle. "Sex puts pressure on you only if you're in the missionary position." The women burst into laughter again. Then more seriously, she says, "I don't worry about being alone. I enjoy being by myself. I did the dating scene. Been there, done that. I don't see any real drawback to being single."

"The hardest part for me is money," says Rita. "I don't make that much, so it's a real struggle living on one salary. One of the reasons I'd get married again is to have more money. He wouldn't have to have a lot; maybe just matching my salary so we could have a house or get a bigger apartment. I lost our house when Larry died and I had to move into a tiny apartment."

Doris excuses herself for butting in. "I forgot something really important. For me, the biggest problem is that I really, really, really want to have at least one child. Some women can have a child by themselves, but I know I couldn't—emotionally or financially. So that clock ticks very loudly for me."

"I feel the same way!" exclaims Bunny. "I want a child *badly*. My cousin, who is 39, adopted a little girl from Korea. She got tired of waiting for a man. But I'm like you, Doris; I couldn't do it by myself."

"I guess I'm real lucky that way," says Margaret. "I decided when I was 16 that I didn't want kids. So I never had to deal with the clock."

"I definitely want children, but I definitely want a husband too," says Bunny. "I know I just said there were advantages to not having a man, but even so, I want one. I'm sick of all this dating around. I do it a lot, even with men I know aren't good husband material. It seems I always have to have a boyfriend; I never go more than a few months without one. I'm sure I do this because I really like to be held. That is the very worst thing about being single for me. I love curling up in bed with a man."

"It's been years since I've been with a man sexually, so thank goodness for my close friends," Alysha says. "I think I pick my friends by their hugging skills!"

Doris grimaces. "I can't imagine going a long time without sex. No one touching me! It's too much a reminder of all I went through with my ex. That's the main reason I go out with so many men. How do you manage, Alysha?"

"You get used to doing without it. Time helps. After a while, you even stop thinking about it. Menopause also helps."

Rita grins. "It must be an open secret among women that we prefer hugging to intercourse!"

There's a rumble as the women agree, everyone except Doris, who says, "That doesn't fit for me, Rita. I love sex!"

Margaret adds, "I like sex, but if I had to give up sex or cuddling, it would be sex, no question. Yet, I occasionally do get horny, real bad. I haven't learned how to turn off my sexual feelings like you do, Alysha."

No one else seems ready to pursue that subject, although by the end of the three hours, they will have talked at length about dealing with sexual feelings when there is no available partner.

Instead, Rita veers off in a new direction. "I just can't figure out what I'm doing wrong. I've read all the books; I go to singles dances and parties. I even respond to singles ads. Shortly after starting to date again, I learned about the 'nine-second rule.'"

Several women smile in acknowledgment, but Margaret asks, "What's that?"

Doris explains. "A man decides if he likes you in just nine seconds. So you have to look just right, say the right thing, 'cause you have only those nine seconds to get his attention."

The discussion evolves from how to "dress for success with men" to all the things women are doing or not doing that keep men from being interested in them. The list of self-blame is extensive. I interrupt to inquire, "How do you understand what has just happened here? Earlier, you were talking about what's wrong with men that they don't know how to relate to and talk with women. Now you're blaming yourselves for not meeting interesting men."

There's a long silence. Doris finally breaks it. "You know, society says you should be married, and if you're not, there's something wrong with you. I guess I buy that."

I push my point. "Are you even aware of how you flip back and forth between blaming yourselves for not meeting appropriate men and believing that men aren't doing their part in order to have a healthy relationship with you?"

"At times I can see that," Rita answers, her voice soft and hesitant. "I know it's not a black-and-white issue. I *do* want to be married again, but only if it's going to be a good relationship. I've had bad ones galore. I guess it's just easier to blame myself."

Margaret picks up on this. "Society teaches us we can have everything we want in life. But we don't want to admit that that's not true; we don't have control over some things. We have no control over meeting non-schmoes."

Alysha, who has become the wise woman of the group, concurs. "It's like we look around and say, 'We can't control these men out there; we can't change them, so we internalize like Rita, or like you did in your second marriage, Doris. We blame ourselves. We listen to these people who tell us to be nicer, less choosy. But that gets us nowhere. We have to remember we have no control over meeting the right man for us. So, we need to just go about living our lives—with or without a man."

Rita shakes her head. "Maybe, but I do think there's something wrong with me because I don't get asked out a lot. Well, a number of men have asked me, but I wouldn't go with them. I'm not that hard up! I've only dated a few men in all the years since Larry died."

"I've dated all those men you've turned down," Doris chuckles. "I listen to you having dated only a few men, and I think that's nice. You're particular, you're not going to waste your time on self-centered, insensitive dolts."

"And you're both here today, still single," notes Margaret. "Guess it doesn't make much difference."

Alysha turns to Rita and chants in a singsong voice, "You're too choosy; you're too choosy!" The group laughs.

Bunny, missing the humor, says, "I don't think I'm *too* choosy, but I am choosy." She pauses, realizes what Alysha is doing, and grins.

Alysha looks at Bunny and gently adds, "Of course you should be choosy. But most women spend more time picking out a car than a man. They're very choosy then, looking at style, color, type of interior, and that's just a car! And as Karen just pointed out, some women may be so glad to just have a man that we don't think in terms of whether it's the right one for what we need and what we want.

"That's true," Margaret nods. "But the sad truth is that as we get choosier, as we get healthier, we only want a man who is mature enough not to be afraid of a strong woman or of intimacy.

"That narrows our choices considerably."

"That's one reason I'm not interested in men now," Alysha continues. "I've seen what's out there and I've just given up thinking I'll meet a man. If you take all the men in the world, 98 percent of them are not worthy of my time and effort."

Bunny quickly jumps in with, "That leaves 2 percent for all the rest of us to share!" Again, the laughter among these five strangers is filled with warmth and mutual understanding.

It's Not As Simple As It Used To Be

The contradiction—it's my fault versus men aren't doing their part—is pervasive, yet it's so subtle, most women aren't aware how they bounce back and forth with these ideas. As Bunny later says, "It's simpler the way it used to be, blaming ourselves for why we aren't married."

Like you, these women grew up in a world that valued marriage. Studies from the mid-1950s showed that 96 percent of American adults married and that 80 percent believed the people who chose not to marry were "sick, neurotic, and immoral," according to G. Gurin, J. Veroff, and S. C. Feld in *Amer-*

icans View Their Mental Health (Basic Books, 1960). Those who remained single did so for negative reasons, such as hating men or feeling ugly. They bore the stigma of "old maid" and "spinster."

While there were exceptions, most girls growing up during this period were raised with the expectation they would marry. The question was not "if" but "when." Oh, they might have a career as a nurse or teacher, because they needed to be prepared. As many women repeatedly heard, "In case something happens to your husband, you'll have something to fall back on."

Things began to change with the sexual revolution of the 1960s. Helen Gurley Brown's *Sex and the Single Girl* (Random House, 1962) was like a Molotov cocktail thrown into society, breaking old taboos and urging women to be more assertive, to own their competence, and to keep their options open for marrying or not.

During the 1980s and 1990s, numerous research studies showed that women were choosing to remain single for positive reasons, such as more opportunity for personal development, increased freedom, and acknowledgment of their homosexuality. For those women who never married, like Margaret and Bunny, the societal changes absolved them from the spinster stigma. They could pursue careers if they so chose, and they were freed from the pressure of *having* to be married for the sake of being married. Married women like Alysha, if they could financially support themselves, were choosing to leave oppressive or abusive relationships.

Things have changed, but let's not kid ourselves. We still live in a society that, at worst, is still prejudiced against singles or, at best, has a cultural ambivalence toward them. True, there are more services for and recognition of singles than ever before: social events, religious groups, newspapers, and trips solely for singles. Along with these, however, is a resistance to accepting singles on an equal par with other—that is, married—adults. The norm is marriage, as evidenced by the phrase "marital status," one's status relative to being married. You have it or you don't.

One Stereotype Is No Better Than Another

You were raised with the stigma of being single, but now, as an adult, you have to live with a glamorized image of a single woman. According to a study by David Atkins, published in the *Journal of Broadcasting and Electronic Media* (vol. 35, 1991), the media helped fuel society's move from stigmatizing single women to glamorizing them. Today's television shows present the single woman as professionally successful, independent, and unencumbered by life's demands. The "Our Miss Brooks" of the 1950s has been replaced by the Mary Tyler Moore of the 1970s and the Murphy Brown of the 1980s.

While the old image doesn't describe most single women, the modern one is equally unrealistic. Not all single women are professionally successful; not all are even career women. Glass ceilings, sexism, racism, and classism affect women equally—with or without a husband. And not all single women are free to do what they want, unencumbered by life's demands. They too have aging parents, bills that must be paid, clothes that must be washed, cars that need repairing, and other responsibilities.

Television, recognizing it had swung too far in glamorizing singles, gave birth to Ally McBeal in the 1990s. She is a single woman who is desperate to be married. While some people see this as a throwback to the 1950s, another interpretation is that now both sides of modern women's ambivalence about being single are represented in the media. Unfortunately, both sides aren't represented within the same woman. These stereotypes are also colorblind, as evidenced in Terry McMillan's delightful and touching *Waiting to Exhale* (Pocketbooks, 1992).

Any way you look at it, single women are presented as one-dimensional: either loving their single life or hating it. Have we merely swapped one stereotype for another? How do we move beyond stereotypes to understand the complexity of feelings women have about being single?

It's Not So Black And White

In the past two decades, most books written about single women present either a black or a white perspective. Bookshelves are filled with advice on how women can attract men and how to live a full life without them. While most of these books have ideas that are useful, none grapples with the full complexity of women's feelings about being single—the pros *and* the cons.

Make a list of your own pros and cons of being single. Now, compare your list with the one below, a compilation of the more frequently mentioned issues from both sides. Should other items be included here—in either column?

Advantages	Disadvantages
not being responsible for others	lacking companionship
being able to do what I want when I want	not having someone to love
having peace and quiet	having to depend on myself for everything
having freedom and independence	missing having someone to share my time and interests
not having to answer to anyone	not being the focus of anyone's love and attention
making my own decisions	feeling lonely sometimes
controlling my own money	having no one to join in spontaneous activity
not having to clean up after others	
not having to impress or worry about others	being responsible for my financial support
being able to focus on personal growth	lacking affection, physical contact, sex

You probably noticed that some of these advantages can also be perceived as disadvantages, and vice versa, depending on your perspective at the moment. For example, being able to make decisions without having to compromise or consult with anyone has a distinct allure, but the flip side is that you're having to make all the decisions by yourself.

Margaret has a clear understanding of the interplay between the advantages and the drawbacks. Early in the discussion, she states that the best part of being single is "having the freedom to work on me—who I am, where I'm going in my life. I can pay attention to my personal growth without having to deal with a husband and marriage problems." Later in the discussion, however, she adds, "The worst part, though, is that there's a part of me that will get developed and grow only within a relationship, a part of me that I'll only know in context to someone else. So, if I remain single, there's a part of me that will never get developed."

Most single women get satisfaction from their work, have close friends, are settled in their home life, with interests outside of the office. They don't pine for a man, yet—at times—they do hunger for one. They can't easily be boxed into any one stereotype of a single woman because there simply isn't one.

Who Is The Single Woman?

A single woman is "unmarried." The negative prefix implies a deviation from the norm—marriage. A single woman, then, is often described by who she *isn't*. Yet, if we extended this to its logical conclusion, this means a woman is a "non-man"; a short person is "non-tall."

Eliminating the deficit term "unmarried" still leaves confusion, for the phrase "single woman" encompasses a variety of circumstances. It refers to women who want to marry and who want to remarry, as well as those who don't want to be married at all but wouldn't mind living with a man in a committed relationship. It includes women who are dating, who wish they were dating, and those, like nuns or lesbians, who have no interest in dating men at all.

The phrase includes 20-year-olds as well as 70-year-olds. Parents, and women without children. Those who call themselves single and those who call themselves divorced or widowed.

Consider this example, which illustrates the confusion. When filling out a credit card application, Marsha, who has been living with Lenny for 15 years, must check the box labeled "single." Louise, on the other hand, who has been separated, but never legally divorced, from Martin for those same 15 years, must check the box labeled "married."

According to the 1991 edition of *Black's Law Dictionary,* a single woman is defined as "unmarried"; single also applies to a widow, and sometimes even to "a married woman living apart from her husband."

When Did You Become Single?

If you used to be married, you know when you became single again. But it's not so clear when you first became single. Other than marriage, society has no rite of passage for transitioning from adolescence to adulthood. Nor is there a socially recognized distinction for moving from being a young single to an adult single. This may explain why so many women feel as Valerie (whom we'll meet in Chapter 10) does when she says, "I feel like I'm still 17, when I'm more than twice that! You're brought up to be a responsible person, and being a responsible person means being married and having kids, right?"

Why Are You Single?

Because of society's one-dimensional stereotype of singlehood, many women feel compelled to have a simple explanation for why they have not found a man they want as a life partner—with or without marriage. And the simplest one for a single woman is always blaming herself. Certainly, others have plenty of explanations for you: you're too choosy, you're too fussy, you don't give a man a chance, you're more interested in your profession, you're afraid of intimacy, etc.

Later in the study group's discussion, Margaret talks about the pressure she sometimes feels to explain why she's single. "When my neighbor invites me to dinner, she always talks about my being single. True, she's an older woman, so I suppose it's excusable, but I still hate it. She'll ask, 'Why hasn't some nice man snatched you up?'"

Bunny grimaces. "It's not just old people who ask that. I got into a conversation with a woman in the grocery store recently while we waited in a long checkout line. She has three young children and has been a stay-at-home mom. Maybe that accounts for her comment. When she learned that I had never been married, she smiled and said, 'Oh, you've taken the career path.' Ugh! I just hate that!" Bunny emphatically tells the group. "I didn't take one path or the other. Marriage just hasn't happened."

"My biggest pet peeve," offers Doris, "is when people tell me I'm too choosy, that's why I haven't remarried. Why do I, or any of us, need to have an explanation?"

My reply to the group is, "Consider this: You may be single because *you just are!* There may not be a comprehensive, this-is-it reason. Maybe you had personal problems along the way. Maybe you were building your career. Maybe you made some good decisions to avoid certain men. Maybe you've been scared of getting too close to a man. Maybe you've worked hard on that fear of intimacy and now are willing to try, but only with a man who is equally willing to work and try, and you haven't met him yet.

"There are lots of maybes to account for your being single, including chance—not being at the right place at the right time. There's also the ever-cited statistics that there are fewer men in your age bracket who would be interested in meeting you.

"Then again, there may be men who are interested in you, but a far more relevant question is whether you are interested in them. After all, if you've spent years improving your emotional health, you *should* be choosy. You don't just want a man; you want a man who will add to your life. You want a man who is equally willing to take responsibility for making your relationship work. You may choose to *remain single* until you meet such a man, even though you don't choose *to be single!*" Consider the following true story, for example.

Where The Men Are

One evening, as five friends were sitting around deciding where they might go (with the unspoken agenda of meeting men), one of them offered a tongue-in-cheek suggestion. "Before trekking all over town, let's figure out the odds for and against meeting Prince Charming tonight."

The ensuing discussion went something like this.

"How many people live in Manhattan? Maybe 7 million. If half of them are men, that means there are only about 3½ million possible partners. If we figure that we're looking just at those between the ages of 35 and 50, that brings the number down to about 800,000 prospects.

"Now, about half of those are unmarried, leaving 400,000 up for grabs. Only a third of the single men are heterosexual and not already partnered, which leaves 133,000 eligibles. If we eliminate those with serious mental problems, we'd have about 68,400. And we're not even looking at the income side yet.

"Those with an income above $25,000 probably number 19,520—if we're generous. And if we then demand that they be nice, intelligent, and humorous, we're down to 6,003. And we still haven't factored in race or religion for those of us who have a preference. Given all this, there probably aren't more than a thousand men out there who are willing to make a commitment. So why bother going out?"

And they didn't.

As long as you are single, you may be subjected, like Margaret, Bunny, and Doris, to comments from others. But even if you are lucky enough to be spared such remarks, you grew up in a world with a clear message that women *should* be married. The next chapter takes a closer look at cultural biases against your being single.

Messages And
Self-Blame

When I was four years old, my grandparents gave my parents a baby grand so I could take piano lessons. It sat prominently in the living room, and I eagerly played throughout my childhood. I grew up hearing, "It'll be yours when you get married."

Once I was on my own, I bought a cheap secondhand upright piano. Each time I moved, I either paid to have it transported, or I bought another one. It was only when I was nearly 39 (and in the second house I had owned) that it occurred to me I was playing on these clunker pianos while my baby grand sat unused—waiting for me to get married! I couldn't believe I had never thought to question the message, to alter the story.

It took me several days of mental preparation before I broached the subject with my parents. I assumed they would hold me to the original agreement. How ironic: my mother was surprised that none of us had thought about this before; she exclaimed, "*Of course* you should have the piano."

The Trance

This is what some therapists call a family trance. Whole families are guided for years by a single phrase or image: "She's a tomboy." "She's so shy." "The piano will be yours when you marry." Despite the passing years, they forget to question if the image still fits.

Family trances are based on cultural messages passed down through the generations. Most midlife single women have their own outrageous stories reflecting the internalized messages that helped frame their expectations of life as a female, that said their lives would be complete only when they married.

As a result, many women have been covertly, if not overtly, taught, "Even if you are smarter, more athletic, etc., than a man, don't let him know it." Women have forgone a career to get married, or they have avoided a career in a male-dominated field because they were not supposed to compete with men.

Conversely, they chose such a career *because* there was more opportunity to meet men. They have geared their lives to obey the primary message: find a man!

If they are unsuccessful—regardless of their other accomplishments—they may feel they've failed.

Naomi and her mom are caught in their particular family trance. Naomi responded to the message to find a man by marrying her high school sweetheart long before she was old enough to know who she was or what she wanted to do with her life. Two children and ten years later, she got a divorce. Her mother still persistently asks her, however, "When are you going to remarry? Why don't you have a boyfriend?"

"My mother says I am looking for the perfect man," Naomi complains. "She thinks I should lower my standards. If I act dumber, that would help me catch a man. She says the main reason I am still single is that I don't hide my intelligence."

Is Naomi's mother cruel and pushy? No. Her mother is caught in that ubiquitous phenomenon of a family— no, a *societal*—trance. While most adults today would agree that women can live complete lives without a man, they still are entranced by the old message.

As with all family trances, the message is passed along unconsciously. Therefore, it is hard to identify and stop repeating the message that it is a woman's responsibility to find a man and get married. If we were to hear that message said out loud, it would sound ridiculous. Few people would say that a woman must be married to be fulfilled. Yet, this trance is perpetuated in our society.

In an effort to break that societal trance about single women, I have identified nine of the most common messages. Many midlife women have heard some of these as they were growing up. They are not presented in any specific order, nor has every woman heard every one of them. You may have heard some of them, but they may not have affected you. On the other hand, you may have absorbed some without even knowing you have been influenced by them.

Nine Messages About Being Single

1. Find a man.

2. You don't give a guy a chance.

3. If you're too smart, men won't like you.

4. You'll find a man only after you stop looking.

5. It's more important that he like you than it is for you to like him.

6. It's better to have loved and lost than never to have loved at all.

7. You should always look good, just in case you bump into your future husband.

8. As you get older, you get too set in your ways.

9. You're smart to have stayed single (the modern message).

Message #1: Find A Man.

Alice, an Always Single in her late 40s, has her own international consulting business. She laughs as she tells the following story, but her laughter turns bitter before she finishes.

"Looking for a man is like cleaning a bathroom. It's something you should do. No one says it that directly, but you just know that's what they think.

"My mother always asks what I did over the weekend. If I don't mention a man, no matter what interesting things I did do, she is disappointed. I can hear it in her voice. And if I stayed home and watched TV, she says, 'Why didn't you go out?' You know, *she* often doesn't go out on weekends, but because I'm single, I'm supposed to."

We've heard this message since elementary school days, when having a profession was secondary to being married. In college we were teased about majoring in husbandry or going for our M-R-S degree. Today's comic strips like *Momma* and *Cathy* convey essentially the same message, which the humor doesn't disguise: find a man.

Message #2: You Don't Give A Guy A Chance.

This message has several well-worn variations: "You're too fussy." "Your standards are too high." "You're looking for Mr. Right." "You expect too much." "You aren't trying hard enough." And the kicker, "If you really wanted to get married, you would."

The following situation is probably equally familiar.

You've been out with a man one, two, or three times. You decide you don't want to see him again. But when you mention this to someone, you hear, "Why not?" Saying you're not interested, even offering a specific reason ("He has bad breath and dirty fingernails," or "He talked only about himself; he never showed interest in anything I said") doesn't stop the other person from shooting back, "You never give a man a chance."

One day Babs stormed into my office, furious after an upsetting conversation at lunch. She's an Always Single 41-year-old secretary, but she delivered this story through the angry tears of a child frustrated at not being heard.

"If you knew your jeweler had 20 years of experience, would you question his statement that your watch was not fixable or that a stone was an opal? Of course not! He's experienced. He knows his business. Well, I'm experienced, too. I know my business. I've had two decades of experience in meeting men. Maybe I do jump to conclusions, but I do it based on experience. I don't need to go out with a man for months to know if I'm bored, or if he's threatened by me, or if he's totally insensitive.

"In fact, I shouldn't even have to give an excuse for why I don't like a man. I just don't—that should be enough. Why do I have to explain myself? Why is my judgment challenged? What do people think? That I'm some moron? That I don't know whose company I enjoy, or who's a good choice for me?"

If you guessed that Babs is indirectly defending herself to her mother, you're right. Babs's mother loves her and worries about her, but drives her crazy with the way she shows her concern.

It's not our mothers' fault. They were raised within the same societal trance— a woman is responsible to find a man and marry him—and so they're only trying to be helpful when they talk with us about men. They probably have no idea how much their words hurt. But as bad as their direct message is, the indirect one—when it comes to men, don't trust your instincts—is even worse.

Unfortunately, in real life, the opposite is true. Since what men (or women) say about who they are may not be an honest representation, single women *must* trust their gut, relying on their experience and intuition in assessing if a man is right for them.

Message #3: If You're Too Smart, Men Won't Like You.

One day in the middle of basketball practice, my seventh-grade gym teacher suddenly stopped dribbling the ball. "Girls," she said, "if you are better at sports than boys, never let them know it."

Over the years, that message was repeated many times, although not always as overtly. When I didn't graduate with honors from high school, to make me feel better my mother said: "You can be glad you didn't make it. If you had, you might have gotten a higher grade than your brother and that would have made him feel bad."

To her credit, when reminded of this now, she cringes. But the fact is, in the graduate courses I teach to midlife students, 100 percent of the women say they grew up hearing the same message. Yet most of the male students express surprise that their sisters had been taught this. As one man said, "That's really an insult to me!" True—and to female intelligence as well. It's also true that some women have managed to reject the message that braininess or competence leads to loneliness.

But for many of you, even if you profess to have put it behind you, when you take a closer look at your lives, you may still see its impact. You may consciously present only part of yourself to men, for fear of scaring them off. This approach is so ingrained that it may have become automatic. Think for a moment: How many times have you let a man's erroneous statement go by because correcting it might embarrass him? How often have you let a guy teach you a dance step (or anything) you already knew because you didn't want to hurt his feelings? How many times have you pretended to not know how to fix or finish something because you knew the man would feel good doing it for you?

Message #4: You'll Find A Man Only After You Stop Looking.

Married women will frequently tell their single friends, "It was only after I stopped looking that I met Ted [or Bill or John]." The statement has a ring of authority: the married woman repeating it is proof of its truth. In reality, though, there is usually no basis for this belief. This message blames you for not having a man.

In fact, it's far more likely that you'll find or not find the "man of your dreams" because you run into him in a particular place at a particular time in his life and yours, not because you are looking or have stopped looking.

(You did notice, of course, that this message contradicts the first one, find a man!)

Message #5: It's More Important That He Like You Than It Is For You To Like Him.

No matter what we verbally claim, many women do put more emphasis on how a man feels about them than on how they feel about him. Again, we may know our own thoughts and feelings but behave as if we don't. Listen to this archetypal mother-daughter conversation:

Mother: How was your date?

Daughter: I didn't like him.

Mother: But did he like you?

Instead of replying, "What difference does it make, since I don't like him?" the daughter offers no defense, and goes away feeling bad, often without understanding why. But the message from mom is that the man's opinions are more important than her own daughter's, and that the daughter's worth is measured by how appealing she is to a man.

Message #6: It's Better To Have Loved And Lost Than Never To Have Loved At All.

We can decipher several meanings in this message. The most positive one says it's worth taking a risk on a relationship, even if you ultimately fail. But on the negative side, it implies that "a bad relationship is better than none" because it shows the woman is at least *capable* of a relationship. Although most people who send this message are genuinely concerned, what many single women hear is that any man is better than no man. This interpretation is reinforced through society's emphasis on marriage as the norm.

Women may hear that they're successful only if they're with a man. The implied opposite, of course, is that if they're not with a man, they've failed.

Message #7: You Should Always Look Good, Just In Case You Bump Into Your Future Husband.

How many women do you know who "wouldn't be caught dead without makeup," whether they were just going to the grocery store, to the gym, or to walk the dog? Interestingly, though, you never hear a man talk about having to shave and change from his torn jeans and sweatshirt before going to the corner store for the Sunday paper!

Message #8: As You Get Older, You Get Too Set In Your Ways.

The opposite of this observation can be equally true, and if you are at all self-aware, it probably is. As you get older, you become less rigid, and more able to accept differences. In fact, many women are more accommodating with men now than when they were younger. Now you can distinguish between what's really important to you and where you can be flexible. This is not becoming "less choosy"; rather, it's a sign of maturity and wisdom to become more realistic about what is and isn't worth turning into an issue.

Message #9: You're Smart To Have Stayed Single.

Another variation is, "You've chosen the professional route." Comments like these usually come from married women and men with fantasies of how much better their lives would be if they were single. Remember Bunny's story about being in the checkout line at the grocery store? The stay-at-home mother of three probably thought she was complimenting Bunny for having "taken the career path."

While this message seems to be positive, many women experience it negatively. Whether they are single by choice or by circumstance, the fact that they must explain why they are single too often gets translated into self-blame.

Reflection: Identifying Your Own Messages

1. Look over the list of nine messages. Which ones did you hear directly or indirectly when you were growing up? Which ones do you still hear? Have any of them influenced you or had an impact on any of your life decisions? If you answer No, is it possible the ways they have affected your life have been so subtle you might have missed them?

2. On a large piece of paper, list all of the messages you are conscious of having heard while you were growing up. These might also include your parents' "expectations" of you. Some typical examples are:
   Don't be angry
   If you don't have anything nice to say, don't say anything
   Boys don't like fast girls
   You can never really trust others
   Ladies don't . . . (or, conversely, ladies do . . .)

The messages don't necessarily have to relate to being a woman or being single. List as many as you can recall. You may find that over a period of days, your list grows significantly.

3. Try grouping the messages in categories, such as About Boys, or My Intelligence, or Relating to Friends.

4. Look over your list. What patterns do you notice? How have the messages affected your view of yourself as an adult, as an adult single, as a woman?

Self-Blame

Self-blame is a terrible affliction that can infect your self-image. Pretty soon, you turn against yourself, picking at your most vulnerable parts. Self-blame can be difficult to recognize since it comes in many disguises:

It's Enough to Make You Dizzy

Let's Blame Ourselves

Straight from the Psyche

The Downward Spiral

Working Overtime

It's Enough To Make You Dizzy

I am talking with Cindy, a regional representative of a major corporation. She's in her late 30s and has had several long-term relationships, each of which she has ended. She is articulate, perceptive, and has a gift of cutting through to the gist of an issue—which makes the following conversation even more striking.

Karen: Why and how do you understand your being single?

Cindy: That's a tough one. Well, I'm single because I am not finding anyone I want to marry. But, that's just a surface answer.

Karen: Not necessarily.

Cindy: Well, it is for me. It's partly true, but the question really is, Why aren't I finding anyone? I'm single because I don't believe that any man that I want to marry would want to stay in a relationship with me, and I don't want to go through the pain of leaving.

Karen: That's interesting. You think in terms of his not wanting to stay in a relationship with you, not of your not wanting to stay in a relationship with him.

Cindy: I don't think in terms of that except when I'm trying to get out of a relationship. Then I wonder if I could ever really stay with him or not. I do everything I can to make it work; then when I decide it won't work, I get out. I wonder, "Oh God, what if I had married him?" I couldn't have made a commitment to him anyway. I couldn't have done it.

Karen: You identify your being single as your problem—you can't stay in a relationship with men. Yet you say that you work hard to make it work, but something is wrong with him in the relationship, and you can no longer try to work to make it better.

Cindy: There's a twisted thing in my head that says, "If a man really wanted to stay with me, he wouldn't become or be the asshole he becomes that makes me leave."

Karen: So the assumption is that if a man really wanted to be with you, he would behave better.

Cindy: Right. *If* he behaved better, I wouldn't leave.

Karen: It doesn't occur to you that he's behaving as best he can?

Cindy: After I'm out, it does. I look back on it and realize he did the best he could do, given who he was, and I shouldn't have been there.

Karen: But you still then say, "The reason I'm single is because the man wouldn't want to stay with me"?

Cindy: Yes. (Softly) That's interesting. (Silence) That is what I said, and I almost think I would say it again, even though we just had this conversation and I see the contradiction.

Karen: That's fascinating. Why would you say it again?

Cindy: Because, it's the first thing that comes to my mind.

Before guffawing, or while scratching your head, check to see if you use the same convoluted rationalization. If you hear it in a friend, do you point it out to her, or leave her believing that what she has just said makes good sense?

Let's Blame Ourselves

Listen to almost any group of single women talking about men and you're likely to hear some common themes. Too many women, like Cindy, blame themselves for their singleness, using a tremendous amount of creative energy to concoct stories that explain why they aren't married.

Among the physical explanations given by women in my study are:

"My bust is too big."

"I'm too flat chested."

"I'm overweight."

"I'm plain looking and intelligent, a bad combination."

Personality-related explanations are equally self-flagellating:

"I'm too shy."

"I've got no social skills."

"My independence scares men. I intimidate them."

In addition to these, women can usually dig deeper into their past and dredge up an acceptable neurosis that prevents them from getting married. Among the psychological explanations are:

poor self-image and low-self esteem

unresolved conflicts with their mothers or their fathers

their childhood

their inability to trust men who appear interested in them (a variation on
Groucho Marx's "I wouldn't want to join a club that would have me.")

Whatever their mental ability or physical attributes, women can claim *that* is the reason men aren't interested in them, or *that* is what turns men off. (Note that these explanations are spoken in terms of men not being interested in women, rather than whether or not the women are interested in the men.)

Straight From The Psyche

Modern-day women and men seem to be obsessed with finding a psychological explanation for *everything*. As a therapist, I value psychology and understanding motivations behind human behaviors. But not everything has to have a psychological basis. Sometimes, as Freud is quoted as having said, a cigar is just a cigar.

Nowadays, people devise interpretations to explain why a woman remains —or returns to being—single. No matter what a woman says about why she is single, you can always find a psychological explanation.

She says, "I grew up with two brothers and a father I adored."

Society thinks, "That's why she's single. No man can live up to them."

She says, "My father was very cruel to me when I was a child."

Society thinks, "That's why she's single. She expects all men to treat her badly."

She says, "I was sexually abused as a child."

Society thinks, "That's why she's single. She must fear and/or hate men."

She says, "After he left me, I never wanted to be that vulnerable again."

Society thinks, "That's why she's single. She can't trust men."

She says, "We were so happy. His death just about killed me."

Society thinks, "That's why she's single. She won't let herself love again."

No one denies the effect of a good, bad, or absent father, or a good or bad adult relationship. But the fact is, many women who are married have had these same experiences. So these explanations of why you have trouble dealing with men obviously don't explain your not being married.

Some women do have emotional problems that interfere with their ability to establish intimate relationships. Some choose "bad" men again and again, perhaps needing to play out unfinished business with their mothers and/or fathers. But it is equally possible that bad childhood and adult experiences may actually help women *avoid* bad marriages, by heightening their awareness of potential problems and their consequences.

Don't forget too that many women seek therapy to help them overcome the effects of these bad experiences. If therapy is successful, these explanations are no longer valid reasons for someone not being able to have an intimate relationship.

The Downward Spiral

One day I was driving to a meeting in an unfamiliar neighborhood. I hate being late, so I allowed plenty of time. Not enough, though, because I ended up on the wrong side of town!

I was angry and began to cry; a helplessness overtook me. For the next few minutes, while hating myself for not having checked the map, I flashed on how dumb I had been, last month, not to have guessed that my dressmaker would skip the country with my clothes. I felt pangs of sorrow for my "lost dresses." Seeping out of the edges of this grief was a sadness about a professional paper I had written that had been rejected for publication.

What's happening here? I was on a downward spiral, a condition that is sneaky, creeping up on you before you realize it. It may last only a few minutes or half an hour, but it feels like an unstoppable slide. It may start when you feel bad about an event over which you have no control (getting lost). Feeling helpless at not being able to change the outcome (being late) leads to vulnerability. Once it starts, you slide down and down in a dizzying swirl of self-loathing and self-blame.

As in the game of dominoes, the way you feel in one situation triggers off memories of other situations where you had the same feeling. You feel vulnerable, as if your whole life is out of control. The dizzying swirl continues until you find yourself taking responsibility for all the bad things that have ever happened to you. When you're feeling helpless and hopeless, you may hit the bottom point of the spiral, which for single women often is their lack of a man.

From my recalling the rejected paper I slid into questioning what was wrong with me that a friend did not return my calls. From there, it wasn't a long slide into why wasn't I married? I'd be old and single and miserable for the rest of my life. As you can imagine, by this point I was feeling incredibly disgusted with myself, a total failure in everything in life!

What does getting lost in the car have to do with my being miserable for the rest of my life? Nothing, of course. But a temporary emotional moment can feel like a life sentence of self-blame.

For married women, husbands often are the bottom point of their spiral. If I had been married in the same situation, I might have spiraled from being late, to my lost clothes, rejected paper, unresponsive friend, ending with a litany of complaints about my husband. When you are single, though, the downward spiral ends with blaming yourself for not being married.

Working Overtime

Generalizations aren't facts, but they do indicate a pattern. Many women will recognize this generalization: Men externalize blame about relationships and women internalize it, accepting the blame and assuming they should be doing something differently. This suggests why so many women stay in a bad relationship far too long: it's their fault, and they must fix it. In its extreme form, this results in the battered woman who assumes she deserves to be abused for not pleasing her husband.

This internalized female responsibility for making a relationship work is another form of a social trance. Starting in the 1980s, we saw a backlash to this, which put women in a double bind. If they didn't take responsibility for fixing a problem with a man, they were not doing their job as females. If they hung in and kept trying to improve the relationship, their reward was to be labeled codependent or addicted to love.

Thelma Jean Goodrich, Cheryl Rampage, Barbara Ellman, and Kris Halstead, in their chapter titled "Abusive Marriages" in *Feminist Family Therapy* (W. W. Norton, 1988), present an interesting perspective on why some women stay in destructive relationships.

> While men are taught to pursue a career, women are taught to become more and more proficient at caring for others, anticipating and satisfying their needs. For a man, the harder and more complicated the job, the greater the challenge. Do we believe persevering in a difficult relationship is just as worthy a struggle as persevering in a laboratory to find the cure for some dreaded disease? Each may come to no success, but does each receive equal honor for the effort manifest, the loyalty displayed, and the strength invested? Certainly the answer is no if one looks at the response of society; the man will be commended, the woman condemned, despite the fact that she has done exactly what society told her to do (p. 168).

It's an impossible bind: The harder a woman works at making a healthy relationship with a man, the more likely she is to be blamed for not trying hard enough or for trying too hard. (While men may work hard on the relationship, they don't suffer the expectation that fixing it is their responsibility.)

I often ask women why they work overtime trying to keep alive a relationship they know isn't good for them. Their reasons range from "I want companionship and closeness" to "I probably won't find anyone better." Other explanations include:

Resignation: "If it isn't this man, it'll be another man and his problems."

Fear: "I'm afraid of starting over."

Family pressure: "I don't want to deal with my family's reactions to my leaving him—they like him, they'll blame me."

Ignorance: "I wasn't aware it was a bad relationship at the time."

Desire: "I wanted the sex."

Naivete: "I hoped he would change."

Economics: "He helped me financially."

The most commonly voiced reason, though, is hope: these women hope that someday their efforts will help the man in their life grow and become more emotionally available.

The determination, the overtime efforts, that women put into fixing themselves to improve a relationship may be repeated in their efforts to fix the man. When the relationship pays off, the efforts will have been worth it. Unfortunately, many women don't know when to call it quits, how to recognize that they're working too hard toward an unattainable goal.

What many women *do* know, however, is that if they are not meeting men or involved with a man, it must be their fault. The clear implication of the message, Find a man, is *do something!* The next chapter describes some of the ways women attempt to resolve their "problem" of being single.

Do Something!
The Effect Of The Messages

As a result of the messages they've internalized, many single women feel compelled to do something to resolve this "problem" of being single. Not only do women tend to feel responsible for making relationships work, they may also feel responsible for the absence of a relationship.

Skewed Solutions

In theory, doing something, or problem solving, isn't bad. But when you start with the wrong assumption—that the problem is your fault—you're likely to come up with skewed solutions. Let's look at five of them.

1. The Myth of Taking Control

2. Maneuvering Around the Messages

3. Betraying Yourself

4. De-pressing Yourself

5. Ignoring Your Intuition

The Myth Of Taking Control

One day in a therapy group for single women, the seven participants are talking about problems they see that interfere with their ability to have good relationships with men. Elaine and Anna Beth energetically blame themselves for not having had a serious relationship since their divorce. They apparently have forgotten that in the previous session they admitted they hadn't met any men they *wanted* to know better.

Elaine, a 43-year-old mother of three teenagers, who has been divorced for ten years, suddenly bursts out, "Wait a minute!" She notes that they have gone back to blaming themselves, then she continues. "You know, society tells us we have control over ourselves. So, we start looking around. We can't control these men out there. So we internalize and say, 'Okay, I'll listen to these people who say it's my fault; I'm too choosy; I'm too fat.'"

Anna Beth is unconvinced. As an accountant, she usually looks for statistics and facts. Not when it comes to men, however. Speaking with a thick Southern accent, she drawls, "Well, frankly, I'd rather think it's my weight. Then I can do something about it."

Many women feel like Anna Beth. They'd prefer to have the cause of the problem lie within themselves; that way, they have a chance of solving it. The litany goes this way: "Once I lose weight [get over my depression, am not afraid of intimacy, etc.], I'll be ready for a man."

Women are sometimes so intent on finding a personal explanation for why they are not married that they end up describing themselves as "defective" or as having some problem. Elaine explains the logic behind this. "If the problem lies within you, you may view it as a personal failure, but at least you can tell yourself you have a chance to fix the problem."

Using the "fix-it" strategy, many women bring to therapy the problem they have decided needs fixing. With this skewed mindset, therapy becomes part of a self-improvement plan that can last until a woman meets a man. But at that point, depending on the course of the relationship, one of three things may happen.

1. If the relationship develops, a woman may say: "You see, all that work paid off. I'm healthy now."

2. If the relationship doesn't last, she has a self-blaming explanation: "I wasn't healthy enough after all."

3. If she doesn't meet a man, she tells herself: "I'm not healthy enough yet. I need more therapy."

I'm always amazed at the mental contortions some women go through to fix this problem of being single.

Sue was widowed in her early 20s; in her late 40s, she enters therapy for the first time. It is the early 1980s, when tennis is the rage among singles. Awkwardly crossing and recrossing her legs, Sue calls herself a quitter because she frequently signs up for tennis lessons but always drops out by the third or fourth class.

As I ask more questions, it emerges that Sue hates sports of all kinds. I then ask the obvious question: "Why are you trying so hard to learn tennis?"

"Because," she replies, "playing tennis is a good way to meet men."

If a problem lies outside your control, and it isn't a personal failure, you are helpless. You have no control over its solution; it's an "illusion of control." People feel better if they can convince themselves they are not helpless. Ironically, self-blame becomes useful, leaving you with the hope that you can resolve the problem. If only you work harder, you'll find the solution.

Maneuvering Around The Messages

What do you say if someone asks, "Are you single by choice?" You may give a clear yes or no without considering how complex that simple-looking question really is. Just because you've turned down a man's offer of marriage doesn't necessarily mean you are single by choice. Although you would like to be married, you turned him down because he wasn't right for you. You can turn this around, though. Just because you say you don't want to get married doesn't necessarily mean you're single by choice. This may be your way of feeling you've taken control of being single when you haven't met a man you want to marry.

Many women don't feel they actually made the choice to remain single, since the two options are not equal. That's why the question can be answered by a no as well as a yes.

"No, I'm not single by choice. I haven't chosen to be single; I just haven't met a man I would want to marry yet."

"Yes, I'm single by choice. I would rather not be single, but I am not willing to date or marry just anyone to avoid being single."

These comments reflect what I hear over and over from my patients as well as women in my study. By saying "Yes, I'm single by choice," you avoid others seeing you as desperate to meet a man. It gets people off your back; they won't try to explain your singleness. You might be considered weird, but you're not "damaged merchandise" that can't find a buyer, to use an image from one woman in my study.

If you say you are single by choice, people will eventually stop asking, "Have you found a man yet?" In addition, this approach protects you against disappointment. If you tell yourself you don't want what you don't have, you won't feel as bad for not having it. It defends your self-esteem in a society prejudiced against singles: it is your choice, not your failure, that you aren't married.

On the other hand, if you say "No, I'm not single by choice," you open yourself to others' explanations of why you are single, as well as their unsolicited solutions. This gives more airtime to those old messages about what you should do to avoid being single.

Betraying Yourself

I can still see Betty's face and hear her humiliated whisper as she tells this story. Betty is a take-charge woman with a high-powered position in the U.S. State Department. She has a remarkable skill in using her sense of humor to put problems in perspective.

One day, though, she sat in my office with tears streaming down her face. She had just returned from her tour of duty at the American Consulate in Pretoria, South Africa, and had run into an old college professor, Dr. Elmira Johnson, who was delighted to see her.

"We've been hearing such wonderful things about you," the professor said. "You're back from overseas; I hear you got all these wonderful awards."

Betty expected to bask in the anticipated praise, when Dr. Johnson asked, "Are you married yet?"

Recounting this story, Betty says, "To my horror, I found myself dropping my head, and in a tiny whisper, responding, 'No, I'm not.'"

This may not seem such a horror to all women, but to Betty and many others, it is. There's shame in letting someone else define your reactions. Betty was proud of her accomplishments and quite comfortable being single. But Dr. Johnson's comment brought back that deeply buried message that all the awards in the world are only second to the biggest one—the M-R-S award. Then, instead of being angry at her professor for dismissing her accomplishments, Betty betrays herself. She gives up her own sense of pride in her accomplishments, letting someone she respects dictate how she feels about herself.

You can betray yourself in other ways, especially in relationships with men. Frances, in the same therapy group with Elaine and Anna Beth, raises this topic. A 50-year-old medical transcriptionist, Frances stares at her lap as she says, "Sometimes I'm so horny and hungry to be touched that any halfway decent man's attention can turn me on."

The women squirm while nodding in agreement with Frances. Then Arlene, a retired elementary school principal, leans forward in her seat and clears her throat. "This whole topic is so embarrassing. Clearly, we all know better." She hesitates, then adds: "I don't know what happens. It's like I'm under a spell. I'm my mature self most of the time, but sometimes around a man, I act in ways that are just plain embarrassing! This is especially true if I feel the man is not as smart or as successful as I am. It's as if I make myself smaller in order to make him look bigger. I tell myself it's to protect his ego, so he won't feel bad. But . . ."

Westy, a 42-year-old hair stylist who hasn't said much until now, interrupts Arlene. "I know what you mean." She gives an embarrassed chuckle. "I not only lose myself, I must lose my memory along the way! Tom calls me about once a month. Now, this man is so opinionated and insensitive, I don't even like talking with him! Why do I go out with him?

"I always come back feeling miserable—and angry at *myself,* not at him. After all, I don't have to spend my time with him. I say I won't do it again, but when he calls, I think, 'What the heck, I've nothing else to do tonight.' I don't seem to remember then how awful I will feel when I get back."

What these three women have in common is their reaction to the message they *ought* to be with a man, and if they aren't, they must *do something.* But their attempted solutions lead to violating their standards and betraying themselves. Because they are without a partner, they must find ways to cope with their emotional and sexual desires. Sometimes, they have a face-off between these needs and their standards.

You do have standards, of course. But do you sometimes compromise them and go out with men, or have sex with them, knowing they are not appropriate for you? Do you later wonder, "What in the world was I doing!"

If that sounds familiar, it may be that those internalized phrases like "You're too fussy" or "You're not giving him a chance" are gnawing away inside you. They may explain why you betray yourself by being with a man you know is not good for you, or humiliating yourself by having sex with a man you don't like.

By having sex with a man they don't like—Frances, just to be touched; Arlene, by adjusting how she presents herself in order to please a man; Westy, by choosing to be with a man rather than being alone (as if those were the only two options) —these women are *doing something*. But what they're doing is damaging to their self-esteem.

De-Pressing Yourself

Noreen is a trial lawyer in her mid-40s. Perfectly dressed in her dark blue pin-striped suit, she stares vacantly out my window. I'm the third therapist she has seen in the past ten years. She is depressed, has been since her late 20s, she says, when all her friends started getting married. After she tells me about herself, I gently say,"You do have reason to be depressed, but not because you aren't married."

Her eyes pull back from the window, intensely focusing on me. "You've been telling me you don't feel satisfied with your life. You hate your job, even though you are good at it, and you don't have any close friends. It makes sense you would be depressed; you're leading a life that bores you."

Many women, like Noreen, have a divided life: professionally, they are very successful, but outside of work, they feel like something is missing. If they believe that what is missing within them can be filled *only* by a man, their personal lives may well be boring. And, if they de-press parts of their personality, if they shape who they are to fit what they think a man wants, they *do* have reason to be depressed. De-pressing your potential is depressing.

If, after having spent so much time and energy looking for a man, a woman ends up without a satisfying career, hobbies, deep friendships, significant life experiences, *or* a man, she has good reason to be depressed.

Some women de-press parts of themselves early on, as young adults. Have you de-pressed yourself through any of these situations?

- quitting college because of meeting or needing to support your husband
- refusing a good job offer because you would've been stuck in a small city with no opportunity to meet men
- continuing to date a particular man who wasn't right for you because you didn't think anyone else would like you

Some women de-press parts of themselves for fear of intimidating men. An overwhelming majority of women in my study said they believe their spontaneity, intelligence, competence, assertiveness, and achievements made a difference in how men saw them. The theme was repeated frequently:

"I've been told I'm too assertive. I'm direct and honest. Men are put off by that."

"It scares them. Guys don't want women who are smarter than they are, unless they are looking for a mother."

"I'm intelligent, have a responsible job, and make money. This makes me inappropriate for 95 percent of the men I meet."

Yet, many of these same women, despite their assertions to the contrary, gave examples of how they reshape themselves, like chameleons, to fit each partner or potential partner. For example, one woman asserted: "I don't hide my competence. I just get the man to talk more about himself." She didn't realize that's just another variation of hiding herself!

Trying to fit into the wrong size shoe causes blisters. And, enough blisters can cause a limp. Unfortunately, when people see the limp, they may think the woman walks funny. They won't understand she's not wearing her own size shoe because a man may be intimidated by her big feet.

The strength you use to keep yourself de-pressed is strength wasted. For years psychiatry has preached that depression is anger turned inward. Many women find it much easier to get depressed at themselves for being afraid of intimacy, or weighing too much, or being a bad conversationalist, than to get mad at the larger forces outside their control—societal trances, prejudice against singles, internalized messages, scarcity of emotionally available men.

Instead of or in addition to being depressed, you may have reason to be angry. But don't direct it at yourself. You may be angry at the way you were socialized. You were promised that if you played by the rules, you would be rewarded with tossed rice, but that promise was broken.

You may be angry at a particular man, or at men in general, for not being able to maintain an intimate relationship. (Don't forget that many men are equally stuck in the gender roles they learned as little boys—roles that taught them not to show their feelings.) You may be angry at your family for reinforcing the belief that something is wrong with you for not being married. (But they too have been socialized to think that way.)

Like many women, you may de-press your anger (along with your competence and other abilities) and protectively turn it inward on yourself. The irony, of course, is that if you directly acknowledge your anger, some people will use that as the ultimate explanation for why you're not married: you're an angry, aggressive woman!

Ignoring Your Intuition

Child: Mommy, I'm still hungry. May I have a cookie?

Mother: You can't be hungry; you've just had lunch.

Child: Can we go see this movie?

Father: You don't want to see that one. How about this one?

Child: I don't want to put my coat on. I'm not cold.

Teacher: You are cold; it's cold outside.

Child: Would you walk me to my bedroom? I'm scared of the dark.

Babysitter: Come on, you're not scared of the dark.

And the trip is not too far from these exchanges to this one:

Adult child: I'm thinking of breaking up with Bill.

Mother: Why would you do that? He's such a nice man.

How innocently adults teach children not to trust themselves, not to believe what they feel inside. It is so insidious, yet after years of having your feelings and beliefs challenged, you may begin to doubt yourself. You learn that other people's perceptions must be more accurate.

In the workplace, most women have gained enough confidence that they hold their own. They can't be easily shaken from their knowledge of a situation. But when it comes to men, too many women deny their intuition, ignoring what their gut tells them about a man.

Woman: I knew there was something wrong with him right from the first time we went out.

Question: Then why did you go out with him, not only a second time, but for several months?

Woman: I told myself I wasn't being fair to him. I wasn't giving him a chance. Maybe I was wrong about what I was picking up.

Question: How often do you later learn your intuition is correct?

Woman: Probably most of the time.

Being aware of who is and isn't a potentially healthy partner means trusting your instinct, listening to your inner voice. Unfortunately, a woman's inner voice often is drowned out by the messages she heard from too many people who told her over the years that she wasn't giving a man a chance. When a woman's perception is constantly challenged, her intuition can become eroded. In time, she may no longer be thinking whether *he is right for her.* She may primarily focus on *becoming right for him.*

What happened to your powers to assess whether this is an appropriate man for you? Whether you will feel good about yourself if you go out with him or not? Whether he is more of a drain on you than adding to your life? After having been single for so many years, after many encounters with men, you *ought* to have a good idea, relatively soon, if this is a man worthy of your time. Knowing this and trusting yourself are part of the advantages of getting older and wiser, of being a midlife single woman.

A Different Solution: The Missing Model

Taking control, maneuvering around the messages, betraying and de-pressing yourself, ignoring your intuition—these are examples of doing something about being single that often result in hurting your self-esteem. Yet, if you think creatively, the requirement to do something may actually open up new options. One option is to think differently about being a single adult.

Social changes have altered our view of life options. Looking at this in perspective, we see that back in the 1940s, Erik H. Erikson opened a new option. In his *Childhood and Society* (W. W. Norton, 1950), he divided life into eight stages, from childhood to old age.

He posited three stages for adults, each with a defining task that, if not met, causes dysfunction. The young adult stage had the task of becoming emotionally and sexually intimate with the opposite sex. If you failed at intimacy, you felt isolated from others. The task for middle adults was being productive, having a sense of accomplishment and meaningfulness in your life. If you didn't accomplish this, you felt stagnated. The task for older adults was reflecting, seeing your life as having some value. If you couldn't do this, you felt despair (see Table 3:1).

You grew up, then, when being single was a transitional phase between adolescence and marriage. According to this life-stage model, if you are single, regardless of your age, you are dangling, "waiting" for your adult life to begin.

The real significance of Erikson's work is that it provided the ground for later theorists to develop a life-stage model that more accurately reflects our society. For example, Gail Sheehy's *Passages* (Dutton, 1976) and *New Passages* (Random House, 1995) describe the midlife patterns for women and men: a revolving cycle of stability followed by a predictable crisis, followed by stability.

Table 3:1 Erik Erickson's Stages And Tasks For Adults

Stage	Task	If Not Met
Young Adulthood	Intimacy	Isolation
Adulthood	Generativity	Stagnation
Maturity	Integrity	Despair

In 1995, Natalie Schwartzberg, Kathy Berliner, and Demaris Jacob opened up another life option. They validated the life stage of Always Singles, for women and men. The authors published their breakthrough research in *Single in a Married World: A Life Cycle Framework for Working with the Unmarried Adult* (W. W. Norton). They identify five stages and their accompanying tasks: 20s, 30s, midlife (40s to mid-50s), later life (50s to when physical health fails), and elderly (between failing health and death). Table 3:2 lists these five stages and their corresponding tasks.

TABLE 3:2 Stages Of The [Always] Single Adult Life Cycle

Life Cycle Stage	Emotional Process
Not yet married	1. Shifting the relationship with the family. Restructuring interaction with family from dependent to an independent orientation. 2. Taking a more autonomous role with regard to the world outside the family in the areas of work and friendships.
The thirties: Entering the "Twilight Zone" of singlehood	1. Facing single status for the first time. 2. Expanding life goals to include other possibilities in addition to marriage.
Midlife (forties to mid-fifties)	1. Addressing the fantasy of the Ideal American family (a) accepting the possibility of never marrying. (b) accepting the possibility of not having own biological children 2. Defining the meaning of work, current and future. 3. Defining an authentic life for oneself that can be accomplished within single status. 4. Establishing adult role for oneself within family of origin.
Later life (fifties to when physical health fails)	1. Consolidating decisions about work life. 2. Enjoying fruits of one's labors and the benefits of singlehood. 3. Acknowledging the future diminishment of physical health. 4. Facing increasing disability and death of loved ones.
Elderly (between failing health and death)	1. Confronting mortality 2. Accepting one's life as it has been lived.

From *Single in a Married World: A Life Cycle Framework for Working with the Unmarried Adult,* by Natalie Schwartzberg, Kathy Berliner, and Demaris Jacob (Norton, 1995), p. 56.

While other life-stage models define people by the "entrances and exits of the children," that is not useful with Always Singles. Therefore, they have targeted other developmental factors for defining life as an adult single. These include relationship with work, finances, peer network, family, and culture.

Each stage has its emotional tasks. The four for midlife include: (1) accepting the possibility of never marrying and not having your own biological children; (2) defining the meaning of work, now and in the future; (3) finding a way of life that fits for you as a single; and (4) establishing yourself as an adult with your parents, siblings, and other family members.

The emotional tasks for later life through old age include accepting your decisions about work and feeling good about your accomplishments; acknowledging the reality of your physical limitations; and confronting your mortality. The final task is accepting your life as you have lived it.

This life-stage model for adults who have never married provides a map, or guideline, for living in a world without a spouse. Much of it also applies to Single Agains.

Today, with more than 15 million women "dangling" for the first or a subsequent time, with so many adults choosing alternative lifestyles, we need new options for thinking about life stages. We need a comprehensive life-stage model that includes all adults—single, single again, married, heterosexual, and homosexual—and one that reflects today's world of evolving relationships. This is especially significant when you consider the following realities:

Everyone is single at some point in life.

Far more than half the adult population is single one or more times throughout their adulthood.

Except in the case of couples who die together, half of every couple (usually the woman) is single when life ends.

The comprehensive model I propose reflects a life course with many twists and turns (see Figure 3:1). The lifeline moves linearly from birth to childhood to adolescence to adulthood, where it splits into two equally viable paths. Some people move along the Single Adulthood path, while others move along the Married Adulthood path. And since women tend to live longer than men, most end their life as a single adult.

This model allows Single Adulthood to be recognized as both a journey toward marriage as well as a destination in its own right. When single, a woman doesn't know if she will marry at a later age, or, if she does marry, whether she will later divorce or become widowed. She may be single several times and married several times, or she may never marry. Therefore, which path a woman's life takes is only known for sure after her life is completed.

While it is an improvement, this comprehensive life-stage model is still incomplete, because it does not address the issue of when one moves from being a

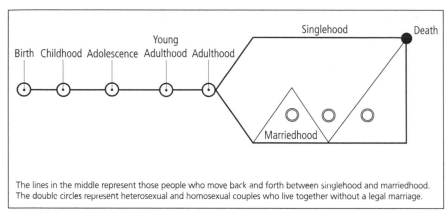

The lines in the middle represent those people who move back and forth between singlehood and marriedhood. The double circles represent heterosexual and homosexual couples who live together without a legal marriage.

Figure 3:1 A Proposed Life Stage Model

young single to an adult single. It does not recognize the cycling of the generations, the different stages that exist for adults with children, nor the unique status of lesbian and gay adults.

Although flawed, this comprehensive model nevertheless provides a framework for society to acknowledge the two equal paths through adulthood and to remove the value judgment that one path (marriage) is better than the other (singlehood). If the societal value judgment were eliminated, it might be easier for a woman to build a single world since she could openly acknowledge the complexity of her feelings about being single. Without feeling shame, she could admit wanting to be partnered or (re)married. At the same time, without feeling hardened and unfeminine, she could admit to loving her singleness and believing a man would add unwanted problems to her balanced life.

Building A Single World

In the same way a couple has to build a married life, a single woman has to build a single life. This may seem unnecessary for Always Singles, since their life position hasn't changed. Yet, as women move from being young singles to adult singles, and formerly married women return to being single, they all need to develop a world that reflects the values and lifestyles of their adulthood, and that meets their needs for a rich and satisfying life—with or without a man.

What does it mean to build a single world? It means you don't put your life on hold until there is a man. It means you don't have control over making an emotionally available man appear, but you can take control of the tools available to you and design the best life you can for yourself. It means accepting that life may not be exactly as you would have wished, but that's true for most people—even married women! It means no waiting, no dangling. It means no self-blame because you have not met a man *you* want to marry.

Building a single world means adapting to change. Like most women born prior to 1960, you may have been raised to expect you would marry and be taken care of by a husband who would protect you, provide you with children, and financially support you. This would make you a fully contented human being. Today, expectations are different, and few role models are available to help you adjust. You need to be flexible, to adapt to living with the ambiguity of not knowing if you will ever marry, or if you do, whether it will last.

For those of you who do not want to be single, you may wonder why you should bother building a single world. But whatever lies ahead, you happen to be single at the present time. *Building a single world doesn't mean making a commitment to being single. It means making a commitment to enjoying your life in the present.*

Think about it this way. You are driving along the highway and find yourself on a different road than you had intended. You have no idea how far it is back to the main highway. You have two choices: you can focus all your attention on getting back to that highway, or you can enjoy the view even while trying to find the right road. Building a single world is like appreciating what the single road has to offer, even while trying to leave it.

Most significantly, building a single life demands thinking for yourself: "What is it *I* want? What is it I need to make my life as fulfilling as possible now?" Many women are not used to choosing what they want for themselves. When they were children, their parents directed their lives. As Always Singles, they may have devoted themselves to finding a man who would shape their lives for them. As married women, they may have pleased a husband, children, in-laws, without thinking what they wanted for themselves. This is why women today need guidelines, tasks, for being an adult single.

The Nine Tasks

Margaret, whom we met in Chapter 1, is reflecting on what it means to be single. "Don't get me wrong. It's not all roses. It's true that most of the time I'm content with my life; I can tolerate the passing moments of longings. But there are times when I get downright depressed. I've noticed there's a pattern to that: when I don't talk with my best friends for a while, or I can't find someone to go to the movies with me, or when things at work aren't going well. These are the times I'm most aware of wishing I had a man."

Margaret also recalls being really depressed about being single when she first moved to her current home. "I had upsetting dreams about my home being washed away. And I was spending so much fixing up this place, I began to worry about money. Oh yes, there also was a time shortly after my dad died. I felt awful about being single, thinking of getting old and being alone. This was a particularly bad time because my sisters and my brother and I weren't getting along well then. I think I pined for a man to help me escape the pain of losing my dad, fighting with my siblings, and of thinking about getting old and being by myself."

What is Margaret really talking about? These issues of intimacy, companionship, groundedness in a home, financial problems, loss of a parent, aging—they're all part of the tasks related to being a midlife single.

Based on my research, I have identified nine tasks for the Single Adulthood life stage. As guidelines, these tasks help women recognize the predictable issues and check how they fare in building and maintaining a satisfying single world. (These tasks, actually, are apt for all adults.) The next nine chapters describe each of these tasks.

1. Being Grounded

2. Meeting Your Basic Needs

3. Making a Decision About Children

4. Enjoying Intimacy

5. Hope for Horniness—Facing Your Sexual Feelings

6. Men! Clarifying Your Thinking About Them

7. Grieving

8. Making Peace with Your Parents

9. Preparing for Old Age

When the tasks aren't met, or when there are temporary gaps in the tasks, as Margaret describes, women may feel depressed or dissatisfied with their lives, blaming it on their being single. In fact, though, the primary cause may be neglecting one or more of these tasks.

Chances are, you already are active in each of these areas. Hopefully, though, assigning names and detailed descriptions to the tasks will make it easier to see the areas where you are doing well, to identify the temporary gaps that need adjusting, and to take action in areas you may have overlooked.

Using these tasks as a guideline for a satisfying single life, you may be pleasantly surprised to see how much you have already figured out on your own. So, congratulate yourself for having forged your own healthy path.

Being Grounded

To build a solid yet flexible single world, you need a solid foundation and good grounding. This represents the quality of being settled within yourself and your surroundings, regardless of whether your love life, or any other part of your life, is as you would wish. It is being settled with what you have even while realistically aspiring to something else. It is knowing the difference between what you have control over and what you don't.

What do you need to get grounded, the first task? To build a foundation? You need to feel you belong in your living space. You need to feel you're part of your neighborhood and community. You need friends and a social life. You need to be doing something meaningful with your career or your avocation.

Being Grounded In Your Home

Can you remember your first adult home—a place where you really belonged? The concept of home has nothing to do with mortgage payments. Your home can be rented or owned; it may be a converted barn or a room in your parents' house. Home is the space you occupy, a place that is *yours*. It reflects who you are and says, "I live here."

Ruth is an energetic, engaging 37-year-old singer who has lived in the same apartment for 12 years. She loves it, even while complaining about its being small. It is sunny and inexpensive. One day she talks about her "cute little apartment." I ask, "Is the emphasis on cute or little or apartment?" She stops to think about that. Before she answers, I add, "If you were living there with a man, how would you describe your place?"

Not needing any time to think about *that* answer, she laughs, "It wouldn't be a cute little apartment, that's for sure!"

Ruth wonders, "How can my same home be cute and little if it is just for me, but not cute and little if testosterone moves in?" What makes the difference, she finally concludes, is that "cute and little" is sufficient for her as a single woman, but if she were living with a man in the same space, it would feel more substantial.

A man's home is his castle; why shouldn't a woman's home be her castle too, with or without a man? When a woman gets married and moves into a home with her husband, she doesn't let the 50 percent divorce rate prevent her from unpacking her things and settling in. Whatever may happen later, she makes the place as comfortable as she can. You have the same obligation to yourself.

Owning Your Own Home

Some women are clear that home ownership is not and will never be right for them. But for many women, owning your own home can be a declaration of status, a rite of passage. Do you say you can't afford to buy? Loads of financial books are filled with ideas for buying without a down payment. Home ownership sometimes takes more ingenuity, legwork, and motivation than it does money. For many women, the real issue has less to do with finances and more with how they see themselves and their family's image of them.

For example, what would your mother say if you told her you were buying a house, townhouse, or condominium? Would it be similar to or different from what your father would say? Would your married sister be jealous because she didn't buy a house until she had been married for several years? Would your grandparents think you were being frivolous with your money, or worry you might scare off a man who thought you were too independent? Would your friends think you were flaunting your money?

Reflection: Owning Your Own Home—Telling Others

Imagine a conversation where you tell each of the important people in your life that you are buying a house or a condominium. Think about where you would be when you tell them—your home, their home, at a restaurant? Are they sitting or standing? What are their facial expressions? What are they *not* saying but you know they are thinking?

Try to picture how they actually see you: A little girl playing house? A grown woman moving into spinsterhood? A poor thing who might as well get a house for herself because she will never have a man to buy it for her? Be as intuitive as you can in imagining each one's response. Be aware that this exercise may make you sad or angry.

Once you have faced the concerns of the important people in your life, it is easier to face your own hesitations. Here's another exercise. Be honest with these questions; at the very least, take note when you want to avoid a question.

Reflection: Owning Your Own Home—Talking To Yourself

Block out a period of time to sit in a comfortable place where you can relax and think. As you ask yourself the following questions, pay attention to which answers come quickly and which ones take more thought. You may want to write out your answers so you can reflect on them at some later date.

1. Are you old enough to own your own home?

2. Are you worthy of having your own home?

3. Can you picture sitting in your home?

4. Can you picture how you would spend your evenings?

5. Can you imagine inviting your parents/siblings/grandparents to dinner in your home?

6. What would be the best part about owning your own home?

7. What would be the worst part about owning your own home?

Were there any surprises? Any insights? If you didn't trip over any of the questions, perhaps you've just gotten into the routine of your life and have forgotten to think about making changes. Maybe change is scary.

Think about whether the important people in your life have any effect on your decision to buy a home or not. Now, consider how your self-image would or would not change if you were to become a homeowner.

The point of these two exercises is not to convince you to buy property. It is to help you learn more about your own decisions. Are they well founded? Are you letting others unconsciously make decisions about where you live? Understanding these issues will help you feel more grounded.

Living Alone Or Sharing Space

Whether you rent or buy, you may want to think about the pros and cons of living alone. Living alone offers such advantages as privacy and independence. The advantages to living with one or several roommates include built-in companionship and shared expenses. A number of living arrangements combine the advantages of both choices. For example, you could buy or rent by yourself; you could buy or rent with one or several others; you could buy by yourself and rent extra rooms to others. Far too often, women live by themselves because that is what most people do. They haven't consciously thought about which living situation is best for them at a given point in their lives.

Some women decide to live with their parents for economic or logistical reasons. Like most decisions, this choice has several pros and cons, which are demonstrated in the following example.

After a long and nasty court battle, Sue's ex-husband won custody of their seven-year-old son and moved across the country. Sue was depressed and felt she had failed as a mother. When her parents suggested she move back home with them, she started packing right away.

Any move should be well considered, not one made by others or while you are feeling helpless, depressed, or defensive. Moving in with her parents made financial sense, and Sue needed her parents' tender loving care, but unfortunately she didn't discuss the boundaries with her parents.

For instance, would she take all her meals with them? Would she have a curfew? What would they expect from her? While she didn't have control over her husband's leaving her, she could have had control of her living space. Instead, she relinquished it to her parents.

Owning The Space Between The Walls

Sue moved back into her childhood room. She had no idea what to do first—get a job, get a new driver's license, unpack, change her mailing address? Her parents were very understanding. They knew she was still in shock, so they walked her through the first few months.

Six months later, Sue is less depressed and has a semblance of order to her life, albeit a temporary one. She has begun therapy, has a part-time job to bring in some income, and is deciding whether to go back to college. She talks and writes regularly to her son, and they are planning their summer vacation. Sue decides to continue living with her parents until she can afford her own place, which she realistically knows won't happen for a few years.

Whether you are living with roommates or parents, you need to decide how much of the space is yours, to decorate and use as you please. Even if you can't afford to buy what you want, you can still make the space "belong" to you. Having the furnishings you want—be it a sofa, rugs, or wall decorations—is important for feeling grounded. If you can't afford your first choice, improvise with your second or third choice. This is what makes the difference between visiting and feeling settled.

Sue finally decides to take charge of her surroundings. The room is still set up as it had been when she lived there almost 20 years earlier. She rearranges the furniture and replaces the decorations from her teen years with items that reflect who she is now. Because she doesn't want to take money from her parents, she paints the room herself; she buys a bedspread, rug, and sheets from a secondhand store. She hangs up photos of her son and pictures he has drawn for her. She converts her childhood room into an adult's room, her home.

Always Singles and Single Agains who have their own apartments or houses often deprive themselves of furnishings they want. They complain they do not have the money or space. They say, "Someday I will get that dining room set I have always loved."

For Always Singles, that "someday" may have less to do with the amount of money in the bank than with the marriage certificate. For widowed Single Agains, that someday may be delayed out of guilt over buying things he would have loved, or using his life insurance money to buy something he couldn't have afforded. For divorced Single Agains, like Sue, that someday may be related to feeling helpless, having given away their personal power. Although you may not have the life you would have chosen, you do have a choice as to how to handle the life you have.

Yet another excuse, which rarely gets voiced aloud, lurks behind these others. "I can't buy the CD (or rocking chair or cookware or whatever) because if I get (re)married, he may already have one." Even a non-superstitious woman may be wary of pushing her luck, thinking, "If I buy it, it might jinx me so I won't get married."

You may scoff at some of these comments, but every one of them reflects those societal messages to single women that we discussed in Chapter 2. If you hear your voice in any of these comments, try asking yourself, "What would I be doing differently about my living space if I were happily married?" Then, use that as a guide for making the space around you belong to you now, as a single adult.

Laura, an Always Single 35-year-old woman, beams as she tells this story. She has a full and contented life. A few years ago she bought a townhouse, long before any of her single friends became homeowners. She has enough money to travel and buy what she wants. Yet, she felt a low-grade sense of deprivation and didn't know why.

Then one day it hit her. She had watched her friends get married and receive gifts that she wanted—items associated with weddings. She decided that while she couldn't take control of finding an appropriate man, she could take control of owning these things.

"I had always dreamed about having a china set when I got married. So, I decided to stop doing without just because I was single. It was real awkward, but I walked right into the department store and registered my pattern, along with all those happy brides-to-be.

"When the saleswoman asked about my upcoming wedding, I took a deep breath and told her I wasn't getting married; I just wanted the set. I secretly grinned at the woman's embarrassment, but felt so proud. Then I told my family and friends about the china pattern I had registered and that that's what I wanted for all future holidays and birthday presents."

Many Single Again women must deal with the same issues. When they return to singlehood, they may notice that their furniture, CDs, and linens don't reflect who they are. They may have been chosen to please or meet the expectations of their husband, parents, or in-laws. For all singles, part of being grounded in your living space is meeting your own expectations, assessing what you have and making sure it reflects who you currently are.

Reflection: Assessing The Space Between Your Walls

With pad in hand, walk around your home, one room at a time. Look carefully at everything: from the floor and everything on it, up the walls and everything on them, to the ceiling. Note when you smile, frown, or feel indifferent. Are you seeing things you've not noticed for years? Jot down the items that make you frown, or things that you know are no longer your taste, or spaces that are empty that you have ignored.

It may not be feasible to change all the things on your list that you don't like; you may not have the money. On the other hand, there may be things that can be changed with more ingenuity than money. Whatever you do, at least you are paying attention to what you have outgrown or ignored.

Location Of Your Home

Another aspect of being grounded is knowing where you want your home to be. Periodically, news stories report which cities have more single men. But these rankings don't distinguish between eligible single men and those who aren't interested in a female partner, such as gays, priests, men already in a committed relationship, or men who wouldn't be an appropriate partner for you.

Where you live *is* important, but not because of men. Some cities are more accepting of singles and are more comfortable with them, while others are clearly geared for couples. If you have a choice about moving, you need to think about job potentials, of course, but also consider if the city fits you. What is the city's personality (bustling vs. laid-back), political climate (conservative vs. liberal), geography (inland vs. coastal)? Does it have a community or neighborhood that fits your lifestyle, where you can feel some camaraderie with your neighbors?

Part of what makes for a contented life, with or without a husband, is a gratifying job, a compatible environment, and good friends. Unfortunately, when women are unhappy with where they live, they may blame it on the absence of a partner rather than on the incompatibility of their personality with the location—the city as well as the neighborhood—of their home.

Being Grounded In Your Neighborhood

Do you know your neighbors? Do you feel a part of your community? Many women buy their own homes, take in their garbage cans, rake their leaves, and chat about the weather with their neighbors across the proverbial fence. But they may be more likely to know what happens in their community by reading the local paper than by participating in the neighborhood.

Why do you need your neighborhood? A basic human need is to belong, to feel a part of a group that cares about your existence, where your presence makes a difference. Feeling like you belong counters existential loneliness. It is too simplistic to blame your dissatisfaction with life and a feeling of emptiness on your lack of a husband. While a husband might help, his absence is not the sole cause of those empty feelings. (Ask your married friends.) Often the real cause of loneliness is feeling empty, feeling ungrounded in your own space, and feeling disconnected from the immediate world around you—feeling like you don't fit in.

An Adult World Requires Participation

When you were a child, your life myopically focused around you and your family. As you get older, if that focus doesn't change, you may continue to feel like a child. Feeling a part of the adult world requires participation in it, *as an adult.* Adults have interests beyond their immediate family; adults become part of other families—neighborhood and community families, a friendship family, and a work family.

As part of your neighborhood family, you can participate in cleanups, block watches, recycling. You can become active in local politics, services to the less fortunate, Scouts, civic organizations. The activity itself is less important than feeling that the people who live on the streets around you are part of your world.

If you are not very involved, what reasons do you give yourself? You're too busy? You have nothing in common with them? In a moment of self-truth, ask yourself: Have you even considered getting involved?

Do you worry that if you were to get involved, it would only make you feel worse about being single, seeing all those neighborhood couples and families? If so, ask yourself a different question: Can you imagine that getting involved could make you feel more connected and less lonely?

Being Grounded In A Social Life

When women talk about being lonely without a man, they may in fact be talking about the loneliness that comes from not having a full and embracing friendship network. When women are content with their lives, they may wish they had a partner, but they don't necessarily dwell on his absence. Therefore, to feel grounded in your present life (as opposed to living for the future), you need a rich social life. This might include convenience and activity friends, married couples, and male friends. (Intimate friendships are important enough to warrant a separate task, which is discussed in detail in Chapter 7.)

Convenience Friends

These friendships are based on mutual needs, such as those shared with neighbors or the mothers of your children's friends. You may not confide in these people, but they are very much a part of your life: taking you to the doctor when your car is broken, going grocery shopping together, etc.

To return to Laura: She lives in a new development of two-story townhouses. Even after being there for several months, she knew very few of her neighbors. She hadn't met the people on the right, but had seen the young couple coming and going. To the left was the Tonti family, with their four children, three cats, and a black Labrador retriever.

"When I moved there, I had high hopes of making good friends, but as the months went by, I realized I never saw anyone. There were no other single people, at least as far as I could tell. One day I was feeling so depressed and lonely, I said, 'What the hell,' and knocked on the couple's door. I introduced myself, said I was new and wanted to meet my neighbors. They introduced themselves and were obviously thrilled I had come over.

"While talking to them, I got the idea to invite them for a picnic the following Sunday. Their reaction was so rewarding that I knocked on the Tontis' door. A commotion of people and animals greeted me. Before I knew it, I had planned a big event. As it turned out, each family brought some stuff and we had a great time—adults, children, animals. It's been two years now, and we've instituted a ritual—one gathering each season. It's just great.

"But the best thing that has come out of it is a real sense of belonging. I don't socialize with them (although I've met some good friends through them that I do go out with). We all have keys to each other's homes; not to come and go, but for emergencies. We do the 'I'm baking and just ran out of eggs; may I borrow three?' routine. If I'm running to the drugstore, I might call and ask if I can pick up something for one of them. And when my battery died last month, Robert took me to the garage to get a new one.

"When Elena Tonti told me that her kids' school wanted to start a block watch, I got actively involved. That evolved into a group of neighbors from the entire development wanting to petition for recycling pickups. If anyone had told me I'd be a civic-minded homeowner, I would have laughed, but here I am. Who knows, I may run for our neighborhood council next year. There are still very few singles my age, but I can't tell you how great it is to feel like I'm really part of this community. You can quote me, if you want, and tell other women, it's *great*. You really feel like you belong to a larger family."

Socializing Or Activity Friends

Another category of friendship are the women with whom you may spend most of your free time. You may not want to share personal feelings with them, but they fill an important place in your daily or weekly social activities. You may have separate friends to go to the movies with and others you hike or play cards with. Your socializing friends may or may not know each other.

Married Friends

Remember Margaret from Chapter 1? Commenting on her friendships, she says, "I have a number of married friends. Sometimes I get together with them, just as a couple, and sometimes I bring my married and single friends together. It all depends on the activity, what we're going to be doing."

The old adage "Two's company, three's a crowd," or the phrase "the fifth wheel," are relics of the past. Many single women have found friendships with couples to be rewarding. Friendships with couples who have children offer participation in a family life, good friends, and perhaps even the opportunity to become a godparent.

Male Friends

The popular movie *When Harry Met Sally* questions whether a woman and a man can be friends—without sex. The following dialogue between three women captures the same discussion. Can a man and a woman stop their sexual relationship and remain friends? Can a man and a woman, with no history of a sexual relationship, be friends?

> Woman #1: John wants to break up with me but asks if we can remain friends. He's got to be kidding!

> Woman #2: That's a good way of making male friends. I have lots of male buddies that I once dated.

> Woman #3: I never dated Bob, but he's one of my best friends. I can't imagine my life without him.

In her recent study, *We're Just Good Friends: Women and Men in Nonromantic Relationships* (Guilford, 1997), Kathy Werking looked at these very same questions. Building on others' previous research, she conducted in-depth interviews of what she called "cross-sex friendships." She met, separately and together, with pairs of nonsexual friends. She acknowledged the limitations of her study since her subjects were primarily young, Caucasian, middle-class, and heterosexual. However, her results offer some ideas worthy of consideration.

". . . Cross-sex friends can care deeply for one another—in many instances 'love' one another. This love, therefore, is not synonymous with romantic love. Rather, it is a love rooted in mutual respect and symmetrical rights and obligations—in short, friendship." Cross-sex friendships can offer comfort, companionship, "equality, affection, intimacy, loyalty, trust, and reciprocity." In addition, they offer a "window into the world of the other sex" (p. 161). Having a male friend—a close, intimate friend or an activity friend—can help you better understand your lover, coworkers, fathers, brothers, and other men in your life.

What is it that makes male-female friendships work? For one, these friendships need clear boundaries about sex, whether spoken or just understood. Will or won't there be sex? The question is superfluous when the man is homosexual. If the woman isn't sexually attracted to the man, he may acquiesce in order not to lose the friendship. (The same is true if the woman wants to be sexual and the man doesn't.) When that happens, either the desire fades or the sexual tension goes underground; to acknowledge it might destroy the friendship.

When there has been a sexual relationship, and the woman knows the man cannot meet her emotional needs, she may prefer to turn it into a friendship because she still enjoys his companionship, as we saw with Woman #2.

On the other hand, if the woman decides the man is not appropriate as a partner, having him as a friend might feel like deprivation, a constant reminder of who he isn't, or what he can't offer her. As woman #1 says, "What attracts me to a man is his ability to be emotional, to share his feelings. If he can't do that, I have no interest in spending any time with him—as a lover or as a friend. If he can do that, I would be sexually attracted, and therefore wouldn't be able to just be friends! So for me, male friends are not an option."

When single women are friends with a married or partnered man, sexual boundaries become especially important. They can be maintained by meeting in public places, not spending too much time alone, avoiding extended eye contact. Another safeguard is to meet the male friend's partner or wife; this removes the mystery and secrecy.

Having males as friends may be easier for women with brothers, if they are used to hanging out with males. It can also work well for women who lost or never had a brother or father. Woman #3 says, "Bob is more like family than anything else. I'd never want to get sexually involved with him; he's like my adopted brother."

Werking found that the male friends often had characteristics women didn't admire, such as no professional ambition, poor money management, living an unstable adult life. Woman #2 talks about one such friend, Tom.

"He's a real good buddy, but we'd make awful lovers. He might like it, but I know that would be the end of our friendship for me. He just isn't what I'd want in a partner. He'd drive me nuts real fast, or I'd learn to hate him, but he's perfect as a friend. Actually, I get the best of Tom and don't have to worry about all these other things."

Based on Werking's study, it does seem easier for younger women to have platonic male friendships than for midlife women. In high schools today, males and females pal around together; in college they are roommates. For a young woman not ready to be sexually active, she can have male companionship without the sex.

There may be fewer midlife cross-sex friendships because our culture has no established guidelines, few role models, and no language for this nonromantic type of friendship. So, adults must improvise.

True, some friends do succumb, as Werking says, to "society's assumptions about male and female relationships," and fall into sex. Many others find ways to "transcend" this, however. As one of Werking's interviewees proffered, "You can always get another boyfriend. You can't replace a friend."

Although Werking's study is significant, it still leaves unanswered the question of why some women can and some can't have nonsexual male friends. One factor that hasn't yet been pursued is a woman's testosterone level. Does that affect her ability to have male friendships? Is her having a low sex drive or being menopausal relevant?

If you can have male friends, consider yourself lucky. If you can't, don't blame yourself, and don't try to push what won't work for you. There are plenty of potential women friends out there.

Being Single Means More Planning

Margaret usually works evenings, but Thursdays she is free. One Thursday she calls Barbara, eager to spend time together over dinner or at a movie. Regrettably, Barbara already has plans. Undaunted, Margaret calls Marilyn, who's tied up babysitting for her granddaughter. Pam isn't home, and Eileen has to work. After the sixth call, Margaret no longer cares about going out. She settles into her favorite chair with a book, the TV remote control, and a cup of tea.

Is she lonely? Does she worry that no one likes her? There is no doubt she will be alone tonight, and being turned down by six friends is a lot of rejection, whatever the cause! This type of evening could set off a downward spiral (see Chapter 3). Margaret could feel abandoned by everyone; she could be angry at being single, reasoning that if she had a husband, she wouldn't have to go through this. She could also be saying, "What a shame it's so hard to find people to do things with on the spur of the moment."

What makes the difference in how Margaret reacts has less to do with the situation than with how she is feeling about herself at that moment. If she has had a bad day, she may feel lonely or even unloved. If not, she might be disappointed, but still enjoy being alone.

The reality is that being single requires much more social planning. Some women schedule time each week to go through the newspapers, finding interesting activities and events, then calling friends to join them. In the absence of the built-in social life implied by marriage, you have to work harder at making your social life happen. Having a variety of different types of friends, women and men, is therefore especially important for single women.

Some women say, "I don't need friends; I like being alone," or "I enjoy my own company." Being comfortable alone doesn't have to exclude reaching out to others, though. It is important for a woman to enjoy being with herself, and it is equally important to get together with people whose company you enjoy.

Reflection: Social Life Chart

Do you assume your social life would be very different if you had a husband? If you answer yes, then try this exercise. On a large piece of paper, draw a vertical line down the middle of the page. On the left side, list things you imagine doing socially if you were married. Would you be having small dinner parties at home, going dancing, getting together with his friends from work?

Then, on the right side of the paper, next to each item, write ideas of how you could handle each one of these imagined social events *now*, in your current single life.

Friendship Family

A friendship family is a nucleus of caring friends among whom you experience different levels of intimacy. These are the people in your life with whom you come together and develop a history. Supportive friendship families are a wonderful asset and a stabilizing force for single women. When women don't have a husband or partner, when they don't have or aren't close to their nuclear family, they can still meet some of their relational and emotional needs by creating a family of friends.

Rosmond and two friends started spending Thanksgiving together when they were roommates their freshman year in college. By their senior year, they had been joined by two other dorm mates who didn't go home for the holiday. Over the three decades since they've graduated, they have continued getting together for Thanksgiving. Of the original group of five, Rosmond and one other have remained single, two have divorced and remarried, and one is still married to her college sweetheart. The gatherings have now expanded to include spouses, mates, and children. Calling it "Our Weekend," the group gathers from all across the country for an event they wouldn't miss. Few have any other contact during the year.

Similarly, Kate, who has been Single Again for 34 years, has developed a close network of female friends. They are all single, all around the same age, all living in the same city. The level of trust and personal sharing varies among the ten women, with some spending every weekend together while others join in less frequently. Combinations of them travel together, and whichever ones are available spend holidays together.

Eunice comes from a terribly abusive family. After years of feeling alone, she has "adopted" a family. Every summer she vacations with a friend and her husband and three kids. Sometimes, the friend's mother and other relatives join in. Eunice has become a part of their extended family. She has both a younger and an older generation who know and care about her. Even though she has no contact with her own parents, and seldom hears from her nomadic brother, she does not feel "family-less."

Being Grounded In A Career

Do you have a job or a career? You need a job, of course, to financially support yourself, but you need a career too—work that excites you, that gives you satisfaction. (Later in this chapter we'll look at when work is just a job.)

Psychologist Erik Erikson said that in adulthood, being productive and creative are vital for a healthy adjustment. Without a sense of gratification from one's work, there is personal stagnation.

This is about more than just a work ethic. It involves the satisfaction of giving of yourself and seeing the results. As a single woman, you will probably look to your career as a major source of your gratification. Therefore, it is important that your work be fulfilling.

Many women feel satisfied and personally rewarded through their career. The workplace is a setting where they are appreciated, recognized, and valued. They can see they make a difference. They can see things change because of their efforts. Even if they do not get feedback from the boss, they may still reap the gratification of knowing that what they have contributed is valuable.

"Workaholism"

Anything can be taken to the extreme. Workaholism, or over-involvement with work, can be a symptom of dissatisfaction with other parts of your life. Some women find more satisfaction in the workplace than they do outside of it. At work you have tasks to do, people to contact, reports to write. There is always something that needs attention, someone who needs you. When being at home is associated with boredom, loneliness, isolation, or not being important to others, it makes more sense to put yourself where you are useful and valued.

The danger for some women, though, is that work becomes their only source of gratification, of feeling valued. For these women, workaholism has become a substitute for real life. Other women may have a problem setting limits on how much to give to the job; they are unable to say no to or to disappoint an employer. It is easy to do this when there is nothing more compelling calling to you from outside of work.

The Work Family

Along with providing income and a sense of fulfillment, work can also provide a sense of belonging. Do you spend more hours at work than in any other part of your life? Most working adults do. A work family may provide contact with people on a daily basis, people you come to care about as you learn about their lives. This is true to some extent even if you don't particularly like your coworkers. A work family may also provide a chance to develop friendships that grow into real intimacy.

Even if you don't socialize with them outside of work, coworkers are a part of your life. Research has shown that for women, losing a job is painful not just because of its effects on someone's finances and self-esteem, but also because of the loss of the ongoing relationships. Obviously, not everyone is lucky enough to have a supportive and caring work setting. However, you have a right to look for it! If your career is important, but you don't feel at home in your job, perhaps you need to consider a change.

Change can be frightening, but that may not be the main reason why a woman stays in a bad work situation. Some women hate where they work, hate the way they are treated, but can't think about leaving. Some theories of organizational development have concluded that a bad work environment may replicate a bad home environment. When a woman is raised in an abusive family, she may be more willing to stay in an abusive job. She may not realize how she is being mistreated since it feels familiar. Or she may hate it, but can't imagine leaving. People from a non-abusive family, though, can sidestep the destructiveness at work, or refuse to put up with it and change jobs.

Reflection: You And Work

1. Can you recognize:
   if you are being mistreated at work?
   what keeps you from leaving, even though you are being mistreated?
   if your boss is taking advantage of you?
   if your boss is being seductive?
   if you are being paid enough for what you do?
   if you are being treated with respect?

2. Are you afraid to:
   ask for a raise?
   point out an inequity in salaries between you and coworkers?
   document your request for more income, or a smaller workload?
   be as assertive with a boss or supervisor as in your personal life?

3. Consider if there are parallels between your family when you were growing up and your work environment. If so, are you in the same role at work as you were in your family? (See Chapter 11 for more ideas about this.) Have you fled from your family only to find yourself "stuck" in the same situation at work?

4. If you are unclear about any of these questions, you may want to consult your Employee Assistance Program or a therapist who specializes in workplace problems.

5. Remember, your work and your work family should be worthy of your presence and your time.

When Work Is Just A Job

Maybe you have no interest in a career. For you, work may be just an income. You simply want to do a decent job and collect your salary. Your self-esteem is not tied to your work. You have more interest in the hours from five o'clock in the evening until nine o'clock the next morning. If so, then it is important to find areas of accomplishment and satisfaction outside of your work hours.

However, be sure that your lack of interest in a career comes from a positive basis, not from self-doubt about your competence. Make sure it doesn't come from family loyalty, that is, a discomfort in being more successful than your brothers or sisters. Patty, Dorothy, and Gail each have a different approach to thinking about work.

Patty and Dorothy both have three sisters. Both are very bright, competent, and energetic, and they are good problem solvers. Both work in the same office: Patty is a secretary and Dorothy directs the training programs.

Patty is underpaid and overworked and is shown little respect for her efforts. Dorothy is also underpaid and overworked, but she sets limits on what she will and won't do. She is comfortable in demanding respect and is thinking about where this job will take her. Patty sees this as the job she will have for life.

What accounts for their differences? For one, the two women have different personalities. Yet, there are other factors related to their family. Both have three sisters. Patty and her sisters were raised in poverty with a non-abusive but alcoholic father. Two of her sisters are on welfare, and the third never keeps a job more than a few months. Patty has a decent standard of living, has middle-class values, and hopes her son will go to college. Her sisters have no aspirations for a better life.

Patty feels somewhat apologetic that she earns more money than they do, that she has a nice home and car. She underplays her expectations for her son when she talks to her sisters. "I don't want them to think I'm any better than they are." When asked how she would feel if she were to go back to school for a master's degree in business, she explains, "That has to be just a pipe dream. I couldn't really do that. They would resent me. No, maybe it's me; maybe I would feel like I've deserted them, let them down. I want them to like me and still include me. That would make me too different from them."

Two of Dorothy's sisters have incomes and a lifestyle similar to hers. The third doesn't work but is married to a very wealthy man. Striving to move ahead is valued and respected in Dorothy's family. "Sometimes, when I get too complaisant, Janie chides me into a challenge, like the time she said, 'Which of us will get a raise first?' I hadn't even thought of asking for one. So I did. Actually, I don't remember who won that, I just know I felt supported and encouraged to get ahead professionally."

Gail's perspective on life differs from both Patty's and Dorothy's. She has worked in the same shoe store for almost 12 years and has little emotional investment in what she does. "I work to make a living. I have a small house and a car and enough money for the things that are important to me. I don't need much more." What things are important to her? "I spend most of my time at the children's hospital. I have done everything there from stuffing envelopes for a special fund-raising benefit to talking with the kids, to organizing outings sponsored by big business. That's where my heart really is. I also love my garden and spend countless hours puttering around."

Unlike Patty, Gail is not holding herself back because of family loyalty. She has exactly what she wants—a job that pays enough for her to engage in her real passion at the children's hospital.

You too may choose to work just to make a living, while putting your real energy into the things that bring you satisfaction. There should be no value judgment about a job versus a career. The value rests in your using your creativity and abilities.

Thinking Ahead

When we were younger, those of us who are now 40 or older were rarely taught to think of a career, to plan for their future—other than marriage and children. We seldom thought ahead to the rest of our working years, about how we wanted to spend our 40-plus hours a week earning a living.

A few years ago, my friend Cheri decided to take a new job, knowing that it meant she would have to move to a new city and initially take a huge pay cut. She had looked ahead to where she wanted to be in the future and figured the best way to get there was to take what looked like a step backward for a few months.

Most women have not been socialized to think in terms of five-year plans, to think about where they want to be and what they have to do to get there. Yet every professionally successful woman I have met—who had a plan—gives credit to her pre-thinking. And those successful women who have meandered their way to success always advise others not to follow their path; instead, they should "make a plan of their own and make it happen."

Go for it! With or without a man, take charge of what you want in your home life, your social life, your work life.

Self-Assessment

The first task, Being Grounded, involves four key issues. Look them over to see how you are doing in each one.

Your Home

___owning the space between the walls
___decisions about ownership or living arrangements
___location of your home

Your Neighborhood

___finding one that fits you
___finding a way to feel a part of it

Your Social Life

___having convenience friends
___having activity friends
___having married friends
___having male friends
___planning your social activities
___developing a friendship family

Your Career

___avoiding workaholism
___expecting to be treated well in your work family
___assessing if you want to simply hold a job or pursue a career
___planning ahead for your career

For any category that you are satisfied with, give yourself a "star," either figuratively or literally. For any that you still need to work on, think about what needs to be added or changed in order for it to be satisfactory. Then, write your ideas for that category.

If you are stuck, talk with friends or family to see how they handle that task. If you are still stuck after that, consider reading a self-help book, taking a course that deals with the topic, or talking with a professional in the area, such as a real estate agent, an interior designer, a career counselor, a financial counselor, or an employee assistance counselor.

5

Meeting Your Basic Needs

What is the major difference between being married (or partnered) and being single? If you answer, "having a husband," you are missing something extremely important. It's not the presence or absence of a man, it's what happens or doesn't happen *as a result of his absence*. A single woman has the same basic needs as a married one, but—and this is the crux of the issue—she must find ways to have these needs met without relying on a man to meet them for her. This is the second task.

From Morning To Night

What is your typical day like? Do you get up, have coffee, read the paper, eat breakfast, maybe jog? Do you then dress and rush off to work? You may or may not take a lunch break, and then it is five o'clock. Are you finished for the day, or do you work late? How do you spend your evenings—working out at the gym, chatting with friends, watching TV, taking a class? Maybe you read in bed until you fall asleep.

Thinking back on your day, how many people do you actually talk to about something other than the Xerox machine breaking or the results of a business meeting? How many people do you talk to that you also talked to yesterday? Do any of these people know more about you than your job description?

If you are lucky enough to work in a setting with people you like, you may have a continuity of human contact. If you travel, work independently, or work in a large workspace, you may not see the same people each day. You may not have someone to talk to about the intriguing exchange you just had with the homeless woman who sits outside your office, or to ask about your colleague who left early with a severe headache the day before.

Trudy has been a sales representative for the same computer software company for a long time. She's on the road every day, often not getting home until late in the evening.

"Basically, I work for myself; I love it, but there are some drawbacks. For instance, I find it difficult to come home and not have anyone to talk with. Yesterday, I had this wonderful experience and no one to tell it to. I could have called a friend when I got home, but it wasn't important enough to make a special call, especially since it was almost eleven o'clock."

We all know the experience of seeing something and wishing a friend had been there so we could laugh or talk about it together. Think about the special moments you have had, the pearls in your day that passed without further recall.

Trudy recounts this story. "I had forgotten it until I was asked to think about special moments that have passed into oblivion. During the victory celebration after the Gulf War, I hung out at the Mall in Washington, D.C., talking with soldiers in town for the event. Some of these brief conversations were painfully touching as the young men talked about their dead pals or the discomfort of getting recognition for 'just doing my job.'

"That evening, I remember my phone didn't ring at all, and I was so filled with emotions from the day that I didn't even think about calling anyone. By the next day, I was back into my routine, so this became another one of my many unshared experiences. It would have been different if I had a husband, a roommate, or a neighbor I see every day—someone who asks about my day."

Is it important to share these experiences? Sharing may be more than a conversation or mutual laugh. Sharing experiences helps them become part of your history, memorializes them in your vast collection of life's uneventful encounters. Without the retelling, they may fade from memory. And, as my 89-year-old mother says, "Life is a collection of memories."

Sharing is important for the special moments as well as the routine minutiae of your day. Not talking to anyone about them may add to a feeling of disconnection from others. You may assume this disconnection is related to the absence of a partner, but it may have more to do with the lack of continuity of people in your life.

Married people may yawn as their partners repeat stories of their often boring daily events. But the telling is important because of the awareness that someone is listening. It is an answer to the question, "Does anyone really care that I existed today?"

I live alone and often go to bed late. I discovered one of my neighbors is a night owl too. When my dog was alive, I made it a habit to drop by each night when I was out walking Indie. Under other circumstances, Judy and I might rarely have seen each other, but it was so nice to have the same human being to chat with about the day or to complain to about a sore throat.

Lack of continuity of people in your life adds to your sense of disconnection. This is different from loneliness, however, which single women may also feel. As with disconnection, women may assume their loneliness is related to their singleness, but that's also probably not totally true. Everyone feels loneliness at different times, for a variety of reasons.

If you want a man in your life and you don't have one, you may feel a deep loneliness. There's nothing you can do about that. You don't have control over making an appropriate man appear. Loneliness doesn't have to be debilitating, though. You can cut the edge of it, sometimes, by choosing not to be by yourself, by calling or getting together with others. While reaching out to friends won't remove the deep loneliness, it will make you feel more connected, which does ease the intensity of the loneliness.

A wedding band doesn't counter loneliness, but what may is the continuity of your daily contacts, knowing that someone is aware of your presence and cares that you are alive.

Feeling Secure: It's 11:00 PM. Does Anyone Know Where You Are?

Along with the need for emotional connection is a woman's need to pay close attention to her safety and security. This is especially true if there is no one who would immediately notice her absence.

"If I were to drop dead in my bathroom, I probably wouldn't be discovered for days," says Trudy. "If a friend called, and I didn't answer the phone, she'd just think I'm out. If work called, they'd just assume I'd become irresponsible and forgotten to tell them I was out of town."

Years ago, a colleague from New York was talking about one of her clients. Laura jogs daily, but before going out each morning, she calls her friend and gives her the route she'll be taking and the expected time of her return. She calls again when she gets home. That gives Laura the security that if she doesn't make the second call, someone will be worried and will know where to come look for her.

Is that being childish? Certainly not in New York! But perhaps not in *any* city or town. Accidents, not just violence, can happen. Laura could faint or twist her ankle, and no one might come by. If no one knew she was out or where she was, she could be in pain or trouble for far too long.

If you are out of town by yourself and have an accident or die, how would anyone at home find out? Most women think they have covered this issue by leaving their itinerary and phone numbers with coworkers or family members. An itinerary, though, is only useful if home needs to reach the traveler, not if the traveler is in trouble.

Consider making this change in your routine: call in every few days, even if it's just leaving a message on the answering machine. When you go biking or hiking by yourself for the day, let someone know where you'll be going, when you'll be back, and call in when you return.

While some of you may nod your head and say, "Yes, that makes sense," you may also know in your heart that you won't do it. Why? Why are we so reluctant to take extra precautions? Perhaps we don't want to acknowledge the reality that bad things can occur. "If I don't consider it a possibility, it won't happen." Perhaps there's a rugged individualism that says, "I can manage by myself." Perhaps it comes too close to feeling like a child having to "check in" with Mom. But can you imagine checking in for yourself—because *you* care about your safety?

Be honest. After reading all this, will you do anything differently?

Needing Physical Touch

The number one drawback to being single may be the absence of physical touch. Not being hugged or cuddled is a major loss for single women, far more, says almost all research on women, than the absence of sexual intercourse. This was confirmed among the women in the study group we met in Chapter 1.

Psychology has known for years that touch deprivation in infants can lead to "failure to thrive." This means that when children are deprived of the basic needs of physical and emotional contact, they often die. No one, though, has considered the effect of touch deprivation on adults. It is not critical for their physical survival, as with infants, but "skin hunger," as sociologist Ashley Montague calls it, never goes away.

Gertrude, Dolores, and Caroline are three extremely different single women. They are talking about what it is like for them not having physical contact.

When her husband, Bernie, died 7 years ago, 84-year-old Gertrude thought her world would end. She couldn't imagine how she could continue living. Then, as time passed, she established a new routine for her life without him. However, there was one thing she longed for more than anything else.

"We slept close together for 59 years! Whenever we went out, we always held hands. Some days I miss Bernie's touch so much I think I'll burst. Sometimes, I 'accidentally' brush against a man's arm just so I can recapture that warm feeling of Bernie's skin."

Dolores is almost 30 years younger than Gertrude and has had a very different life. Dolores left Martin about 12 years ago. She was so busy with her children and managing her work and home that she had no time or interest in meeting other men.

When her youngest son left for college last fall, Dolores's friends thought she would begin dating. She says: "I don't really care about men. If it weren't for missing the physical touch, I would have no desire to be with another man. Yet, I do miss that. Yesterday, I had a shocking realization: the only person I had touched all week was the doorman. He took my hand helping me get out of the cab."

Thirty-nine-year old Caroline has had numerous lovers over the years but hasn't been in a relationship for 2 years. "I know I'm not the only woman who sleeps with her dog, but how many women do you know who cuddle with them? I wrap myself around Taffy because I like feeling a warm body. I do love holding him, but I sure miss being held." She grins, "I haven't been able to teach him to do that yet!"

Replenishing The Physical Contact

Don't let anyone fool you; there is no adequate substitute for romantic touch. You may experience a deep tactical hunger for it. But along with missing romantic touch, you may not be getting enough of *any* type of physical contact. Do you know how you compensate for its absence?

Some women numb their feelings and deny their need for touch. Some become cranky, rigid, or hardened. Others become depressed without realizing the connection between their depression and their lack of touch. And still others fill the physical void in self-demeaning ways, such as overeating, drinking, or sexual promiscuity.

While you don't have control over finding a man and having your tactile needs met, you do have control over finding adequate substitutes to meet that very basic need for physical contact. You can replenish it in many self-enhancing ways. Hugging friends, being affectionate with children (yours or others'). Taking up activities that involve touching, such as dancing or massage. Pets are another source of ready and willing touch.

One day Dolores told her friends the story about touching the doorman. She was surprised to hear that others felt the same way. One friend said she gets her "touch-fix" from her weekly massage. Dolores decided she couldn't afford the time and cost of a massage every week. "Instead, I now go every two or three weeks. And you know, I can really tell the difference. I don't snap at others so quickly, and I don't have this deadening feeling inside my skin all the time."

Rituals For Singles

"In some ways, my life is no different now than when I was 23," says Gladys. "In these last 20 years, I've been promoted at work, and I have more gray hair. What else is different? I still live alone. Oh yes, I now pay the bank instead of a landlord. But the basic shape of my life is the same."

Janet can't say that. She's the same age as Gladys, but in the past 20 years she has been married, had two children and one miscarriage, lived through discovering her husband's affair, and decided to get a divorce.

Rituals give meaning to your life, marking transitions. So, it's understandable that Gladys, who has not celebrated the life events that traditionally get marked—engagements, weddings, baby showers, christenings—has no sense of her life being any different now than 20 years ago. Despite modern life's greater acceptance of singles, there are no religious, government, or social rituals that specifically celebrate events of the single life.

In Volume 23 (1984) of *Family Process,* family researchers Steve Wolin and Linda Bennett defined rituals as "a symbolic form of communication that, owing to the satisfaction that family members experience through its repetition, is acted out in a systematic fashion over time." Rituals contribute to the "establishment and preservation" of a family's sense of itself (p. 401).

Applied to singles, this means rituals contribute to the "establishment and preservation" of a single woman's sense of herself. Rituals give value and authenticity to singlehood. They mark special events, major life transitions, and even daily aspects of a woman's life.

Wolin and Bennett also found that the *absence* of rituals in families is an earmark of their dysfunction. Does that mean if singles don't have rituals, they are dysfunctional? Absolutely not! In reality, everyone has rituals, at least the daily ones, but they may not be ones you've planned or are even aware exist. For instance, my dog taught me that I had apparently created a ritual for taking her for a walk. Whenever I blew my nose, she would run for her leash.

Because society has no established special event or life transition rituals for singles, you must establish your own.

Establishing Your Own Rituals

When a woman marries, the ritual of a wedding celebrates her entering a new stage of life. What a woman who is waiting for marriage in order for her life to start is really waiting for is a celebration of who she is, a stamp of approval of her life. Without rituals, it *is* harder to feel grounded in life.

Celebrations or rituals that are centered around marriage and children imply these are the "achievements" that get rewarded. But *you* can choose which aspects of your life and your development are worthy of celebration. You can ask friends and family to arrange a celebration for you, or you can plan it yourself. For example, give yourself a party honoring a promotion or salary raise. Create a ceremony for moving from one city to another. Create a ritual for honoring the day of your birth. All birthdays are worth celebrating, but you might create a unique ritual for a specific age, like turning 50. For my 55th birthday, I decided to ritualize the whole year; I celebrated each month with different friends. After your parents die, you may want a ritual welcoming you to the position of being the older generation.

Inside your head you might be protesting: "Oh no! I couldn't possibly plan my own celebration. That's self-centered." But there's nothing wrong with being self-centered or selfish in its literal meaning, "about or of the self." Even the

Bible speaks of honoring ourselves in the verse, "If I am not for me, then who will be?"

Obviously, it would be nice if others thought to honor your life passages; after all, a bride-to-be doesn't have to ask someone to throw her a shower. But the reality is that others probably won't think of it. More important, though, is the question: What's wrong with tooting your own horn? Aren't you worth it? Haven't you earned it? If you think about it, there's probably more reason to celebrate your job promotion than to celebrate your getting married. One is partially the result of luck, fate, or happenstance; the other is primarily the result of your hard work.

What are some of your life events that may deserve honoring? Getting your first mortgage may be worthy of a ritual. Couples have housewarming parties when they buy their first or subsequent house. Although some single women don't think about noting this important step, owning your own home is a measure of a woman seeing herself as an independent person, not relying on a man for her life's direction. It is a way for her to say, "I'm taking charge of my life; I don't like paying rent; I want to own my space." Or: "I'm thinking about my financial future—a home is good equity. My decision to buy is totally separate from the issue of my meeting a man."

Some single women eliminate or put on hold the rituals they enjoyed as a child, saying, for example, "When I have children and a family I will observe that holiday, or light Friday night candles." Why not now? How can you adapt rituals to your life as a single woman?

One of the loveliest rituals I've discovered was two close friends who sent each other a card on the anniversary of when they decided their friendship started. Can you think of other important anniversaries in your life worth celebrating?

In addition to major life events, rituals can be created around your daily life. Meals can be a source of pleasure, rather than one more thing you avoid because you are alone. Dinner can become a ritual for unwinding from your busy day. It can be a time to sit quietly for a few minutes, reflecting and daydreaming.

Start or end your day by luxuriating in the sensuousness of a long hot bath. Or, keep a journal or scrapbook to record your history-in-the-making; have a regularly scheduled dinner with friends; buy yourself flowers once a week. Some women even create a ritual for the first year after their last menstrual period.

Not all of these events are directly related to being single, but they are part of your life as a single woman and therefore worthy of being marked as a special occasion.

How To Create Rituals

Rituals can be complex or simple; you can make them up or adapt existing ones. I've read of one journalist, for example, whose morning ritual begins with stretching and deep breathing, moves to naming three things she wants to accomplish during the day, and ends with throwing her arms open to receive the day. It is simple and takes merely a few minutes.

Rituals all have a beginning, a middle, and an end, regardless of how simple or complex they are. The beginning of a ritual marks the line between regular life and this special time. The middle indicates the essence or the point of the ritual, and the ending brings closure.

When you are about to create a ritual, consider these four steps. Preparation and planning include the design of the ritual. What is being honored and how do you want to have it happen? The people should be considered next. Whom do you want to include, and how do you want them included? Do you want them to be witnesses or active participants? Next, consider where you want the ritual to take place. Is it practical to get there? Should there be any special significance to the location? Finally, how will your guests participate? Will you expect some to contribute more than others, depending on their age, ability, or relationship to you?

Rituals can be used in so many ways. They can help shape and maintain relationships, as in the case of the two women who send each other cards on the anniversary of the beginning of their friendship. Rituals can mark changes and transitions in your life, as for a housewarming, a job promotion, the onset of menopause.

Rituals can be used to help you heal and recover from betrayals, trauma, and loss. A cleansing ritual involving water, good friends, and kind words, for instance, can be important after a woman has ended an abusive relationship or has been raped.

Rituals can be used to express your beliefs and values. And, finally, rituals can be created for no specific reason other than to honor your life and joyful times. (For more ideas about creating rituals, see *Rituals for Our Times* by Evan Imber-Black and Janine Roberts [Harper Collins, 1992.])

Reflection: Rituals For Honoring Your Accomplishments

1. List all of the accomplishments you've had since you turned 30 (or 21 or any other age). This may be difficult. Many single women have a difficult time deciding what to consider an accomplishment. Think in terms of job, friendships, family relationships, personal changes and growth, adventures you've had, and risks you've taken.

2. Next to each one, note how it was honored. If there was any form of a ritual, describe it.

3. For any that weren't honored, imagine what type of ritual you might have created for them.

4. Now, highlight each accomplishment from the past year.

5. If they have not been honored yet, create (at least in your mind's eye) a ritual for each one. Would you include others in the ritual or would it be something you do by yourself?

6. Be generous with yourself and your life's accomplishments.

7. Be creative. Build off of established rituals or start from your own imagination.

Enhancing The Meaningfulness Of Your Life

Some women feel their life is empty and not meaningful because they are not in love with or loved by a man. However, ask a married woman—even a happily married woman—and you'll hear that having a husband is not enough. There has to be more substance, something that feeds you emotionally, spiritually. Men may come and go, and even children, as they grow up, do not have the same place of importance in your life, or you in theirs.

As you assess your life, think about how you fill your time. Do you find your life revolves around work, dieting, exercise, singles events, errands, movies? Does what you put into your free time leave you enriched, or does it make you feel like the proverbial Chinese dinner: full for the moment, but hungry soon again?

Looking For Men

"I arrived in Montreal on a beautiful fall morning for a well-deserved vacation. After registering and unpacking, I went for a long walk."

Heliene is sharing a story that is common to many women, but few either recognize they do this or would admit it out loud.

"As I returned to the inn, I saw the porch was empty except for one man. Walking up the stairs, I noticed he didn't have a wedding ring (I always notice these things), so I decided to sit for a few minutes. I struck up a conversation (I never skip opportunities to meet men), and although he didn't seem interesting, I heard those old messages about my not trying hard enough, so I told myself maybe he had more spunk than he was showing.

"He not only wasn't interesting, he didn't seem interested in me. 'Well,' say those old messages, 'he may be shy and needs to be pursued. He didn't use the pronoun we, so he must be single.' I quickly retort: 'No ring could also mean he's involved with a woman, or he's gay.' The messages snap back, 'Don't jump to conclusions.'

"'Enough!' I grab hold of myself long enough to turn off those messages. For whatever reason, he was not interested in me. Give up. The retreating voices murmur, 'Well, at least you tried.' As I walk inside, I feel real sad. It's as if I have lost a chance at a husband."

That isn't all Heliene lost; she lost her free time, to say nothing of a piece of her self-esteem. She isn't sad at having to struggle with those old messages, just at the loss of a potential man. She isn't sad at having lost the opportunity to enjoy the view, daydream, read, even doze. Instead, she wastes her free time responding to that old message: find a man.

The good news is that Heliene heard the inner voices and tried to battle them. The bad news is that she isn't angry that the messages are inside her head. Those old messages keep her constantly on the watch for opportunities to meet men. There's no vacation from this. She looks for the telltale signs of the man being available: a ring and the pronouns used in his conversation. She finally acknowledges he's not interested in her; yet, far more important, she doesn't heed her intuition that *she's* not interested in *him*. Heliene isn't aware that even on vacation she is working overtime.

What's your image of Heliene? A desperate 32-year-old or a pathetic older woman of 50 or 60? Do you imagine she's a woman with no inner resources to fulfill her life, living a shallow existence? Or is she a woman who is man hungry? If you guessed any of these, you're wrong. Heliene is a successful businesswoman who is a funny, lively 42-year-old with a good friendship network. She's well read, has a range of interests, and believes in taking good care of herself, which is why, even though she basically works on commission, she still took a week-long vacation.

Still, she struggles with the effect of those old messages. No one watching her that fall morning would believe how those voices harangue her. To the outside world, she is independent and self-assured enough to travel alone to another country. Until now, she has never shared with others the old tapes that run inside her head.

Does Heliene's experience sound familiar? How many hours or minutes a day do you spend thinking about men? How often have you tried to lose just three more pounds before next weekend? Do you honestly know how much of what you do in your non-work time is related to men? You know what the politically correct answer is, what you'd tell others. But are you aware of what you actually do in thinking about men? Do you sometimes push yourself, like Heliene, to devote time and energy to see if a man likes you, ignoring your intuition that says you aren't interested in him?

Three women, all in their 40s, are sitting around a table talking about singles parties. That's what they would say they were talking about, yet, are they?

Beth shifts the discussion to clothing. "When I go out, I dress differently than I do for myself. My friend Janie (she's been single forever) calls it marketing; if you want to meet men, she says, you have to market yourself."

Marilyn nods. "It's like the dating version of 'dress for success.' Your friend Janie is right. There's a certain way you have to dress."

"I was really shaken up after my divorce," Beth adds. "I wasn't able to start dating for over a year. And I felt like a duck out of water. I had no idea what getting back into dating was going to be like. I didn't know how to market myself, or what Margaret called 'dressing for success.' I was still dressing like a married woman. But I knew first impressions are important. I knew I was doing something very wrong. I could tell by men's reactions to me, they just weren't interested."

During this exchange, Tammy has been silently listening. Now she leans forward in her chair and almost shouts: "Wait a minute! Listen to what we are saying here!" Her voice tones down as she continues. "You know, after I left Paul, I learned all this too. I never gave it a thought; I just followed what other single women were doing. But hearing you two talk about it, hearing these words coming from your mouths—not mine—angers me. Why do we have to package ourselves up like some gift to get some man's attention, to get him to like us? Who set the rules, and who says we have to agree to do it? You know, we don't talk about how *he* dresses. Do men have to dress for success with us? Isn't the real issue whether or not *we* are interested in a man, not how we dress or he dresses?"

Beth and Marilyn start to defend themselves and their need to dress appropriately for men. Tammy interrupts and says, "What would we have been talking about for the past hour, if we had eliminated the topic of men?"

Tammy asks an interesting question. Some women fall into the *pattern* of talking about, looking for, thinking about men. It becomes a pattern, or habit, when it fills time, is repetitive, and adds nothing new. She raises two poignant issues: women tend to think more about how to interest some anonymous man they hope to meet than about what they want from men. Second, what would women talk about if they ruled out the topic of men?

The women initially feel defensive when Tammy poses that question, but as they probe it more, they realize that talking about men with other women is a form of bonding. By sharing complaints and analyzing men's behaviors, they feel a sense of camaraderie, of closeness. Marilyn adds, "Besides, it's reassuring to hear other women say the same things I've been thinking. It reminds me it's not just my impression. Lots of women feel the same way."

It's important to state a caveat, here. Although women talking about men each time they get together is a form of connecting, at some point, reshuffling the same old conversations can feed women's helplessness and depression.

Body Image Obsession

Food has become the enemy, and deprivation has become a virtue in our society. In the name of physical well-being and fitness, it has become admirable for women to diet and deprive themselves of food. It has become admirable to spend one or two hours a day at the gym. It has become admirable to feel guilty for *not* depriving yourself of food or *not* exercising.

It's not only anorexics and bulimics who have a distorted body image. While an estimated 20 million women have eating disorders, the American culture as a whole is eating disordered, according to Mary Pipher, author of *Reviving Ophelia* (Putnam, 1994) and *Hunger Pains* (Ballentine, 1995).

Pipher cites the results of *Glamour* magazine's 1984 survey crafted by Drs. Susan and Wayne Wooley for their article "Feeling Fat in a Thin Society." Thirty-three thousand women completed the survey. Seventy-five percent of them said they felt too fat, including those who were actually underweight! Ninety-six percent said their weight affected how they felt about themselves. Given a choice between losing weight, happiness in relationships, success at work, or hearing from an old friend, almost one-half said losing weight would make them happier than anything else!

What's the problem if you have a ripple or roll of flesh? Would your life be any different if that ripple were removed? Every year, 80 million Americans spend 33 billion dollars in their attempts to lose weight, and almost every study reports that 95 percent of those people regain their weight and then add some more.

Geneen Roth observed in *When Food Is Love* (Plume, 1997) that after years of trying to reach (and keep) her ideal weight, she finally met with success, only to discover that losing the weight wasn't her real goal. She was more invested in "getting" thin, not in being thin.

"As long as my attention was consumed by what I ate, what size clothes I wore, how much cellulite I had on the backs of my legs, and what my life would be like when I finally lost the weight, I could not be deeply hurt by another person. My obsession . . . was more dramatic and certainly more immediate than anything that happened between me and a friend or lover. . . .

"The wonderful thing about food is that it doesn't leave, talk back, or have a mind of its own. The difficult thing about people is that they do. Food was my love for seventeen years and demanded nothing of me" (pp. 1–2).

Have you ever noticed that horses pulling carriages wear blinders on the sides of their eyes? That's to keep their focus on the road ahead, so they won't be distracted by what's going on to either side. Think about an obsession with eating, weight, and body size as your blinders. What thoughts or feelings are to either side of you that your body obsession distracts you from? Is it feelings about being single, unresolved issues from childhood, questions about your job, a decision about having children, issues with friends?

An obsession is different from an interest. You might like working out, but you don't get upset if you can't get to the gym on a certain day or for a week, or if you can only work out for 20 minutes instead of an hour and a half. You might want to lose weight, but you don't think about it throughout the day, worry about what you eat, talk about it incessantly, or even dream about food.

Nowadays, it's hard to distinguish between an interest in and an obsession about your weight and health. To help, here are some questions that might clarify the distinction for you.

How much of your free time do you devote to dieting, exercising, and thinking about your weight? With so much subtle pressure on women, do you even know *why* you do these things?

Do you really *not* like chocolate, fried foods, or meat, or have you convinced yourself, "It's not good for me"?

Do you really enjoy the health club and jogging, or have you falsely adopted the line, "I *like* to keep fit"?

An abundance of anything can be unhealthy, but occasional chocolates, fried foods, or meat aren't life threatening for most women. Keeping fit is important, but long daily workouts may be more than necessary. When you eat more than you think you should, or work out less than you think you should, can you shrug it off, or do you beat yourself up for "being bad" and "cheating"? Are you one of the many women who really don't care that much, but feel they *should,* so they feel guilty about eating or not working out?

The obsession with weight and fitness that pervades America today has a special meaning for single women who are barraged with the pervasive message, find a man. A woman may say she diets for health reasons or because she doesn't like the way she feels. But internally, those words may get translated into: "It's my weight that keeps men from being interested in me. If I were thinner, more men would be attracted to me." She's not saying if she were thinner, it would help her find more men *she* found interesting. That, of course, would make no sense!

This weight frenzy is fueled by the advertising industry. For example, a few years ago *USA Today* ran a clothing ad that said, "Let sex do the selling for you." Another contemporary ad proclaims, "If you don't watch your figure, no one else will!!!"

In *The Beauty Myth* (Vintage Books, 1990), Naomi Wolf attributes these types of ads to male-dominated institutions that became threatened by women's freedom as a result of the feminist movement of the '70s. An ideology that helped women feel "worth less" was urgently needed to counteract the way feminism had begun to make us feel "worth more."

The higher women have climbed, the harder the beauty myth has had to work to undermine their achievements. The more successful women become financially and professionally, the more the patriarchal business world needs to defuse female power. This is not a conspiracy theory, says Wolf. There's no need for a conspiracy; women willingly cooperate. Focusing on beauty works against female power, by building a "dark vein of self-hatred, physical obsessions, terror of aging, and dread of lost control" (p. 10).

The beauty industry has benefited as women succumb to the myth of needing to meet some ideal image. A 20-billion-dollar cosmetics industry complements a 300-million-dollar cosmetic surgery industry. Keeping women focused on themselves and how they have not yet achieved some required image keeps them from owning and using their full power. Beauty now is seen as a qualification for women's rise in power; hence, women's poor physical self-image and their lack of confidence in their appearance. When a woman becomes obsessed with mirroring the ideal, it diverts her energy from other things.

This is not to say you shouldn't eat what you want, look how you want, have plastic surgery if you choose. Rather, you need to be sure your choices meet *your* needs. You don't want them shaped by the media, the beauty industry's financial strategy, or your internalized messages.

Think about this: If you cut in half the time you spend on dieting and exercising (doing it, buying for it, and thinking about it), what would you do with all the unspent time? What would you do with your free time if you spent less of it thinking about men?

This might create a gap in your days that would need to be filled. Would it be thinking more carefully about your career? Deciding about adopting a child? Pursuing the hobby you never had time for? Reading those books you keep putting off? Having more interesting discussions with friends? Stopping to smell more roses? Learning what other flowers you like to smell? Figuring out what you need to make your life more meaningful—with or without a man?

Creating Your Meaningful Life

When you are 99, reminiscing about your life while rocking in your favorite chair, how do you hope you'll answer those questions about what you've accomplished? In preparation for that day, is there something you need to do now to make your life feel more meaningful?

In talking about her experience after she returned from Montreal, Heliene said, "One of the worst parts of being single is thinking about getting older and being alone, having nothing meaningful in my life."

When faced with this empty space, many women fill it, as Heliene did, with something they know—the message to find a man. It is as if they say, "If only I could find a husband and have children, then life would be meaningful." Pauline knows differently. She did what was expected; she married and raised two girls and a boy. But her husband died three years ago, just after her 50th birthday.

"I've always lived for someone else—my husband, my children. Now, I'm really searching. Who am I living for now? It feels like something is missing. I suppose I'll need to learn to live for myself. I *could* find another man and live for him, but I don't want to do that. This time I need something more meaningful for me."

In time, Pauline has found something meaningful. She started quilting and has developed a community around it. "My quilting friends have really become like a family to me. They are all over the country, so I might spend time visiting with them, meeting them at quilting conventions."

While Pauline brought something new and meaningful into her world, other women may need to give of themselves and their time to others, be it work with children, saving the forests and wildlife, or cleaning the environment.

Many women in their midyears find solid grounding by turning to religion. A woman I recently met told me that after her third divorce and four career changes, she applied to a doctoral program to become a minister. She hadn't considered that this might be related to her turning 49, yet the reality finally hit that men (and financially successful jobs) would not provide that special meaningfulness in her life.

Having the structure and rituals of a religion may provide a sense of inner peace for some women. They may become more involved in their church or synagogue, teaching children or singing in the choir. Adding personal prayer or the awareness of a deity to their life may be the connection they need for a more meaningful existence. Perhaps the popularity of support groups like Overeaters Anonymous and Alcoholics Anonymous is related to this need for a more meaningful connection to others and an appreciation of a higher power.

Some women, though, turn away at the word *God*, while others react negatively to the word "spirituality." Yet, as Robin Carnes and Sally Craig say in *Sacred Circles: A Guide to Creating Your Own Women's Spirituality Group* (Harper, 1998), spirituality simply means "to inspire." It's derived from the Latin word meaning "to breathe." Women need to breathe more meaningfulness, more passion, into their lives. A spirituality group is a self-selected gathering of women who want to understand, explain, and express themselves. Such groups focus on a woman's journey through life and the obstacles to growth. A woman's spirit, the authors say, "animates us" and keeps women connected with themselves, others, and with what they call "the Great Other."

Their book offers a number of ways women can be inspired, using the support of a women's group. It includes practical information for forming and running sacred circle meetings, and for using storytelling and rituals. If we adopt Carnes and Craig's definition of spirituality, then single women *absolutely* need to feel inspired and to breathe animation into their lives—whether or not they have a man. And along with putting activities and relationships into your life that give meaning and enjoyment, you need to limit the things in your life that devalue you.

Doing so will go a long way toward answering the ponderous questions of life. Whether or not you've had a good marriage will only be a part of your life's history. In an overview of your whole life, you will require far more than a man to make you smile with satisfaction at what you accomplished in your lifetime.

Self-Assessment

The second task, Meeting Your Basic Needs, involves five key issues. Look them over to see how you are doing in each one.

Having Continuity Of Daily Contact With People

Feeling Secure
___when local
___when out of town

Getting Sufficient Physical Touch

Creating Rituals
___for major life events
___for daily life

Enhancing Your Use Of Free Time
___assess the time you "look" for a man
___remove destructive uses of your time
___don't use food and exercise obsessively

For any category that you are satisfied with, give yourself a "star," either figuratively or literally. For any that you still need to work on, think about what needs to be added or changed in order for it to be satisfactory. Then, write your ideas for that category.

If you are stuck, talk with friends or family to see how they handle that task. If you are still stuck after that, consider reading a self-help book, taking a course that deals with the topic, or talking with a professional in the area, for example, a security system analyst, massage therapist, nutritionist, personal trainer, religious counselor. Some of these components don't have a professional expert, which means you need to become your own. (Which also means there may be a market for a consultant in these areas, in case you are considering a new career.)

Making A Decision
About Children

Margaret, whom we met in Chapter 1, says: "I'm not bothered by the proverbial clock because I've always known I didn't want children. That makes being single easier for me than for some women."

Like Margaret, some women know for certain that they don't want to be a mother. Others, however, aren't sure; and some know they do want to have a child but haven't decided how or when to make it happen. Making this decision is the third task.

To Be Or Not To Be—A Mother

To outsiders, Sally looks like she leads a contented life. She owns her own gift shop and a beautifully decorated home. She has good friends and is active in her church and community. But, unlike Margaret, she is frantic. She is 38 and desperately wants a child. As each year passes without her getting married, she gets more depressed.

Sally has never considered having a child outside of marriage. This leaves her in the vulnerable position of having no control over her decision to be a mother. She is dependent on some unknown man for something she herself yearns for.

While a woman has no control over finding an appropriate man, she *does* have control over her decision to have a child. When you become angry at a particular man—or men in general—for "preventing" you from having a child, you are abdicating your power and responsibility for your own life.

Are you childless by choice? You may never have thought about it that way. You may have seen yourself as single, without a child, and continuing that way until you got married. Think about your choices, though. Do you want to be a mother, by choice, or childless, by choice? This removes you from the passive position; you decide what you want, regardless of what happens with a man.

The decision to have a child should be unrelated to your having a husband, unrelated to your gender, or your sexual activity or orientation. Everyone—

women and men—needs to make this decision: Do I want to be a parent or not? This decision should be made only after giving serious consideration to the pros and cons of parenting, which may be different for every woman.

Being a single parent is not for the faint of heart. It is stressful and exhausting, as well as enriching and fun. So, it's important to know how having a child would affect your life—not just now, but across a lifetime of changes and uncertainties. This is important to consider because your life situation is bound to change many times between now and when you die. You may be married and still have to raise your child alone because your husband is a workaholic, travels, or isn't particularly interested in parenting. You may decide to raise a child alone, and later marry. You may be married to a man who is equally involved in child rearing, only to have his health fail him, and leave you a widow. You may decide to adopt a child, knowing you can afford child care, only to have a reverse in your financial situation years from now. Life is full of unknowns.

If, after considering the uncertainties of the future, you still decide you want to be a mother, then you need to decide how strongly you want a child and under what conditions. Do you want a child only if you are married? Do you want to have a child by yourself if you reach a certain age with no potential partner in sight? If so, what is that age?

You need to clarify how much and in what way you want a child. Below are some questions that may help you as you think through this serious matter.

Question #1: Do You Want To Be A Parent?

This question obviously needs to be answered first. If you say yes, you want to parent a child, make sure this is your own desire; that you aren't trying to satisfy someone else's—a parent's, a partner's, society's—expectation of you.

If you answer no, you don't want to parent a child, make sure you are not just giving up because you don't have a husband. If you aren't sure how important having a child will be in your life, give yourself permission to be ambivalent. You don't have to have a ready answer. You may eventually decide yes or no, or you may consciously decide to let fate make that decision for you.

Here's the most important part, though. Know that whatever decision you make, there probably will be many days during the rest of your life when you will wonder if you made the wrong decision.

Question #2: Are You Willing To Raise A Child By Yourself?

Do you want a child *only* if it comes with a husband? Do you want a child *only* if it comes with a foolproof guarantee that you will always have this same husband? That he will always be actively involved as a father?

Do you know that even if you are married, you may still raise your child alone? Ask your mother. If you are from a traditional family with its clear division of household labor, your mother may have been married, but she essentially was a single parent.

Question #3: Do You Have The Resources To Be A Single Mother?

You need two types of resources to successfully raise a child—financial and human. Just for the basic necessities of shelter, food, clothing, and health care, children are expensive. According to a report in 1995 by the Department of Agriculture, the average cost for a middle-income family to raise one child from birth through the age of 17 was $145,320. This doesn't include extras like camp, private schools, or college. Also note that many experts feel this figure is too low!

Furthermore, do you have the funds to hire someone to take care of your child while you work? Do you have a large enough home and the income to consider a live-in helper? Do you have enough money so you don't have to work?

You also need human resources for parenting. Are there relatives or friends who will be a regular part of your child's life? Are some of your friends parents themselves? These may be the people who can provide a support network for when you are feeling emotionally overwhelmed as well as when you need child care. Do you have single friends who are committed enough to be a regular and significant part of your child's life? Could you consider a communal home with one or more single parents?

Question #4: How Do You Want To Become A Mother?

If you've decided you want to have a child, you'll next have to determine how to go about it. Listed below are some of the more common methods. You may have already thought of these, but perhaps seeing them in print may help clarify your thinking. Perhaps you'll think of yet another means.

  a. intercourse with a man who wants a commitment to the child and to you but who does not want marriage

  b. intercourse with a man who wants a commitment to the child but not to you

  c. intercourse with a man who does not want a commitment to you or to the child

  d. intercourse with a specifically chosen man without telling him he is the father

  e. intercourse with a randomly picked man without telling him he is the father

  f. adoption of a child born in the United States (for more on adoptions, see below)

  g. adoption of a child born outside the United States

  h. artificial insemination with semen from someone you know

  i. artificial insemination with semen from a sperm bank (for more on this, see pages 85 and 86)

Question #5: What Type Of Contact Do You Want With The Father?

When the father is known, he may not want marriage, but he may want to be an active parent and participate in his child's life. In some ways, this can be an excellent option, if the two adults have a good working relationship. The details need to be worked out legally so that each parent is protected, as well as the child.

On the other hand, some men are willing to give their sperm but do not want much, if any, contact with or responsibility for the child. In this situation as well, it is important to legally protect yourself from future difficulties in case he should later change his mind about his involvement with his child.

Do be cautious about using a man's sperm without telling him the baby is his. You may think it the best way at the moment, but with so much litigation these days, you may pay the price years later if he comes back and claims paternity.

Question #6: If You Decide To Give Birth To A Child, What Do You Tell Others?

If you decide to get pregnant without being married, of course people will talk. Therefore, you need to decide in advance how you will deal with them. First, what will you tell your parents? Most likely, you will use different language with your mother than with your father. Will they be supportive? Initially? Later?

Consider how to present this information to your mother. Be sure to let her know you have given serious consideration to all the facts, the potential problems, and the sacrifices you know you must make. Decide how much of her involvement you want. Initially, she may want nothing to do with your having a child. Don't get too put off by this response. This may not be her final stance. She may need time to get adjusted to the discomfort of your going against social mores. She may need time to figure out how to deal with her friends' reactions. She may need to actually see you with the baby before she can believe it's really happening.

How do you explain your having a child to your father? Stereotypically, he may need assurance that you have considered the financial obligations and have made plans for the baby's future. He, like your mother, may be worried about what others will think. Remember, you didn't come to your decision quickly, so be generous with your parents. Give them time to have a full range of reactions before they settle on how they want to relate to you and your child. Some women are surprised that after an extremely negative or hateful initial reaction, their parents are quite pleased to be grandparents. (Parents may have the same ambivalent reactions to your adopting a child.)

What do you tell others? Some people will be intrusive and ask who the father is. Others may just look embarrassed or disapproving. You can be certain there will be rumors. The more consistent and firm your responses, the more in control of the conversations you will feel.

Gloria learned too late the need to be prepared, even with her close friends. She had divorced when she was in her early 30s before she and her husband had decided whether to have children. Ten years later, still single, and the CEO of a paper product company, Gloria decided to have a child, and became pregnant.

When her pregnancy began to show, she let her colleagues know this was her choice. "I want to be a mother." Her enthusiasm was infectious; both men and women in the office were excited and talked proudly about her brave and independent decision.

When the baby was born, however, these same people began to pull back. Gloria had never mentioned the father, and no one had asked his identity—at least they never asked *her!* One of the crude jokes circulating around the office was, "Gloria's baby will be born with sideburns and a mustache," referring to Paul, a marketing vice president in the company.

Gloria was not prepared for the nastiness and rejection from her prior supporters. In retrospect, it would have been wiser if she had offered a story about the baby's father, whether true or not. Or if she had made it clear she was not going to discuss it.

By saying nothing about the father, her staff made up their own information. The sad result was that her long-time employee and dear friend, Paul, was the brunt of the rumors, which eventually led to the loss of their friendship, a breakup of his marriage, and his changing jobs. As the boss, Gloria survived, but she paid much too high a price.

You Want A Child, But Only Within A Marriage

Sally looks at the six questions and scrunches up her face. "I do not want to raise a child by myself. I'm sorry; I want to be a mother the right way—a husband first and then a child." She sounds anything but sorry. Her voice is defiant as she continues: "I'm not so modern. I couldn't do it any other way!"

This is a knee-jerk reaction, perhaps an expression of fear. There's nothing wrong with Sally wanting a child only within a marriage. The problem is she is not taking responsibility for this choice.

After considering all the options, you may still want a child *only* within the confines of a marriage. In today's world, that's a reasonable decision—financially, emotionally, and socially. It is expensive and physically and emotionally taxing for anyone to be a parent. Add in the social stigma a single mother may face, and there are many reasons a woman may not want to consider a child outside of a marriage.

However, it is imperative to ask yourself the question and to be comfortable with your decision. If you know you want a child, but only if you're married, you can feel good that you are in charge of your life. You have made a decision based on considering your choices—whether or not you like your choices. Once you have chosen this direction, you have two options.

One option is that you do everything possible to find a husband. The intensity of your wish for a child, the intensity of your rejecting other methods of having a child, means you *must* find a man.

If you are lucky, you will find an appropriate partner. Under the pressure of finding a father for their yet-to-be-born child, though, some women adjust their expectations for a man. They are willing to settle for less so they can give their child wedded parents. Sometimes, on some level, they know the marriage won't last. Even so, this may not be a bad decision. A woman wants a child, needs a husband, chooses a decent man, and the marriage may or may not continue. She has taken charge of her life, given what is available to her.

Unfortunately, some women who choose this option lose too much of themselves in the search: dating very inappropriate men, and putting themselves in demeaning situations. If they don't find someone they want to marry, they end up feeling worse about themselves. They not only lose hope for a child, but also their self-esteem, viewing themselves as a failure because they did not find a man.

The second option is to continue living a full, satisfying life, hoping you will find an appropriate man. You will be active and make yourself available, thus increasing your opportunities to meet a man. You may or may not meet a potential husband, but you can feel content that you have taken responsibility for your decisions. You don't want to raise a child by yourself *and* you don't want to compromise what you need in a husband. It would be a loss not to have a child, but no more than the loss of being with an inappropriate partner.

Neither option is better than the other; there is no right way to do this. Either decision can be the right one for you if you think it through carefully.

Sally will have difficulty with this task of taking charge of her decision about a child. She is not childless by choice, nor is she willing to make the choice to have a child. She is adamant about wanting a husband first, and is actively looking. However, she persists in blaming her childlessness on the absence of a man rather than on her choice about how to have a child.

She says, "That's only playing around with words," but she can't see how she has abnegated responsibility for her choice. The end result—no child without a husband—is exactly the same, but she might feel a bit more empowered, less embittered, and less like a victim if she were to take control of her decision. Otherwise, she continues to blame men, or blames herself for not finding a husband, and then turns her anger inward. Living with her de-pressed anger, she'll be depressed and resentful that life has been unfair to her.

Barri has dealt with the question of having a child quite differently. At 45, she has come to grips with not having a child. "It's the only thing in my past that I never got around to doing." This is a woman who makes things happen—in her life and in the lives of others. She is professionally successful and active on the boards of state and local organizations. She has been a foster mother several times.

Reflecting on her choice, she says: "I always thought I wanted to be a mother. I must not have wanted it enough, though. I have a friend who had artificial insemination, so I certainly could have pursued that. I guess I was sort of fatalistic. I never used birth control; I just figured one day I'd get pregnant."

Would Barri do things differently if she were young again? Perhaps, perhaps not. Although she never saw the six questions listed above, she must not have wanted a child outside of marriage badly enough to make that happen. Unlike Sally, she accepts responsibility for her childlessness, although she feels a deep loss for the child and the family she never had.

You Don't Want Children

All women, but especially singles, should take their time and make a well-considered decision about parenthood. Ask yourself, "Do I choose to be a mother, or do I choose to be childless?"

Personally, I am indebted for my choice to a client I saw back in the '60s, when married women had children because it was expected of them. One day this woman guiltily cried out: "I never should have been a parent. I never thought about it; I just did it." While responding to her tears, I heard bells going off in my head. "Oh, I don't *have* to have them." I was 27 years old and felt very relieved. Although I loved children, at that moment it was clear to me: I didn't want to be a mother.

People often assume I have no children because I'm single. When I was younger, I always corrected them. I wanted people to know I was childless by choice, that my decision about being a mother was separate from the issue of my being a wife. Women who do not want children may cause others to be uncomfortable, not knowing how to respond. For example, if you want a child, but only within a marriage, friends can offer sympathy that you are childless. If you want a child and go ahead and have it, they can talk about your being "so modern." But if you simply don't want a child, they need an explanation. Saying you don't want to be a parent, or you don't want to raise a child, is not sufficient. They assume you must have a problem: something from your childhood, or your selfishness.

Saying you don't want a child because you had a bad childhood is too simplistic an explanation for such a complex issue. Many women who suffered through childhood traumas want and have children and are good mothers. Your decision about having children needs careful consideration, based on your past together with your ideas about your future.

Although my decision happened within seconds, most women struggle with the question for months or even years. Some make a definitive decision when young, and then as they turn 40 or feel the onset of menopause, they doubt themselves. This is a normal reaction to your developmental changes. Major birthdays and menopause are times for reassessing your life. Hesitation about your decision at this point may only be temporary. Accept the doubt and consider your options. You may find within a few days or weeks that you've reasserted your first decision. Or, you may be ready to make a new one.

Unable to be definitive, some women allow fate to make the decision for them. If you are having difficulty with this decision about children, consider seeking professional help. It's an important question that deserves your full participation.

The issue is about choice, not competence. I used to feel compelled to explain why I didn't want children, but I never really knew. Almost 30 years later, though, I am certain my decision was the right one for me. Make sure yours is the right one for you.

You Want A Child

If you're considering raising a child by yourself, take strength and encouragement from the countless women who, through unforeseen circumstances, have become single mothers. Single parenting is doable and rewarding. It holds obstacles and difficulties, as with all of life's ventures. But if you have the emotional fortitude and energy to get through the hoops of having your child, you'll certainly be able to manage all the issues of raising one!

"I did not choose to be a single parent," says Jody. "I was single, and I chose to be a parent. Certainly, I would have preferred to be a married parent." When she was 36, Jody decided that if she were not married by age 40, she would have a child by herself.

"Actually," she explains, "it wasn't quite so simple. When I was in my early 30s, I used to say I'd have one by myself if I weren't married by 35. When I turned 34, I moved it up to 36. When I was 36, I decided I could go on doing this forever, so I settled on the absolute outer limit of age 40. Suddenly, or so it seemed, I turned 39. Nothing had changed my mind, though, especially not the bad relationship I had just ended."

You may already know how you want to go about becoming a parent. If you don't, the following sections contain some ideas on each method to stimulate your thoughts. If you are still unsure, you may want to consult a professional.

Adoption

If you are considering adopting a child, you need to educate yourself about the process. The first step is to think about what you want in a child. Ask yourself what age child do you want and from what nationality. What will you accept? How flexible will you be?

"Agencies can place any parent with a child if the parent is flexible," says Ray Battistelli, director of Adoption Resource and Education for Single Parents, headquartered in Silver Spring, Maryland. Adoption exchange organizations like ARESP can walk you through the sometimes tortuous steps. These are not adoption agencies; they do not bring a child and willing parent together. What they can do, though, is provide information, get you in touch with adoption agencies, and offer support groups and educational classes.

The fact that most big cities have organizations specifically devoted to helping single women adopt a child suggests a growing acceptance of adoptive single mothers. Prejudices do exist, however, which you should be prepared to face. For instance, heterosexual married couples usually have priority for newborns and Caucasians. It is much easier for singles to adopt an older child, a child with special needs, a high-risk minority child, or a child from another country.

At least four ways to go about adopting a child are available to you. There are public adoption agencies, like state and county social services or human services. There are private nonprofit agencies, like Catholic Charities and the Datz Foundation. Independent adoptions are arranged outside of an agency. These are legal in most, but not all, states. With these, it is best to work through an attorney who specializes in adoptions. Then there are many organizations that arrange adoptions of international children.

The cost of an adoption can range from free (public agencies) all the way to 20 to 40 thousand dollars. If you adopt a special-needs child, you may get a monthly financial subsidy.

Martina, a woman with two adopted children, offers this suggestion for finding an adoption agency. "First," she says, "stay away from adoption agencies if at all possible. Take a class [such as those offered at an adoption exchange organization] to learn more about the process, including things often overlooked, such as travel expenses and possible contact with the birth mother. Then, talk with at least five people who have adopted within the last three months. Ask them who they used and what their experience was. Third, contact the agencies they recommend." She adds, "If you contact an agency first, they'll try to convince you to do the adoption with them, their way."

If you are not fortunate enough to be able to consult with other adoptive mothers, you can find adoption agencies through the Yellow Pages, under Adoption Services. In most cities, this is not a small section. Remember, though, you are calling for information. If you don't have a good feeling for one agency, trust your gut. Call others, shop around.

Jody recalls the beginning of her journey in mothering. "I had no idea how to start. I didn't know anyone who had ever done this. In preparation for my 40th birthday, I opened the Yellow Pages. Boy, was I surprised to see how many listings there were! I called about half a dozen before I became so overwhelmed I almost gave up. During one call, though, there was a really nice lady who told me about an adoption exchange organization that could help me.

"Don't forget, during all this time, I'm also working 40-plus hours, dealing with my sick mother, and trying to keep some semblance of order in my life. Now, with the perspective of a few years, I wonder why I didn't give up long ago, but I'm awfully glad I didn't!"

Adoption is not an easy road, especially going it alone. Jody got involved with a group who provided the emotional and concrete support she needed. They sponsored educational classes to prepare her for the adoption process and the home study.

Home studies, which are conducted by a social worker, are a preliminary step for initiating an adoption. They can cost anywhere from a dollar to 15 hundred dollars. It is important that you have confidence in the social worker. Therefore, interview the person in advance and don't be shy; be sure to ask if that person has any hesitation about placing a child with a single woman. While an agency may have an open policy, a particular social worker can make it difficult. Since state laws may vary, it is also critical to ask about the time frame a birth mother has for changing her mind after the adoption has been completed.

As we heard from Jody, it can be a trying and lonely ordeal. ARESP Director Battistelli concurs: "Don't try to go it alone. You need a support network, but don't be too surprised to find your network shifting." Friends who were initially supportive may begin to pull back once you have the child. Some may be threatened by your gumption; or they may withdraw their support when they see you spending more time with your child.

The process can be long and frustrating. Be prepared to bump into many unhelpful and discouraging people, as well as many who want to be helpful and encouraging. If you give up, you may be saying you do not want a child enough to exert the amount of effort it will take to deal with the bureaucracy.

Artificial Insemination

Potential sperm donors are carefully screened for their intelligence and their physical and emotional health. They must have a favorable family health history; they can't have any drugs in their system; and they are tested for venereal diseases. In addition, they are asked to abstain from sexual activity for 48 hours prior to each insemination.

The donor, usually a college student, produces specimen by masturbating in a private room at an approved insemination clinic. This semen is inserted into the woman's reproductive tract at the time of ovulation through one of three methods. Her doctor selects which is most conducive to her medical condition. There's about a one-in-four chance that a pregnancy occurs on the first cycle. Insemination often requires five or six cycles. If still unsuccessful, a new donor is used. The success rate for most artificial insemination programs is 70 to 80 percent.

Even though artificial insemination is not a new medical process, the legal implications (such as social vs. biological paternity) and social ramifications are still muddy. Psychologists have not given sufficient thought to whether inseminated children will have identity problems because they do not know their biological fathers. Might the children have problems, knowing that others may have been born from their same gene pool? How could they be sure they weren't marrying half siblings? What are the genetic implications if they unknowingly marry one such sibling?

None of this is reason to discount insemination, however. Taking control of your life means being aware of the factors before making a major life decision. Most insemination programs include counseling and evaluation as part of the preparation.

(The information here about insemination comes from The American Fertility Society and The American Society for Reproductive Medicine, both located in Birmingham, Alabama.)

Intercourse

The crucial issue about this choice is your adequately screening the donor. You know how to be cautious, physically and emotionally. You should have information from the potential father about venereal disease and drug use. You want to know enough about his personality to anticipate his reactions if he is told— or not told—of his paternity. (Review Question #5, above, for ideas about the amount of contact you want with the father and how to protect yourself from future legal ramifications.)

You still must decide which of the five ways of having a child through intercourse you want. Some of the options may not be available to you if you don't have a willing prospective father in mind. A number of women have found willing fathers in their homosexual friends; often, these are men who also want to be active in parenting.

Children: Good Grief!

Most people live with a low-grade mourning for important things they wanted in their life but didn't get. For single women this may be especially true around the issue of children. Whatever your decision about parenting, you may experience periods of sadness. Grieving for what isn't, or for what you once thought would be part of your life, is normal. You may grieve over your lost motherhood or over the broken (unspoken) promise that a loving husband and children were indelibly engraved in your future. You may mourn your lost marriage and the loss of your children's father.

This grief does not necessarily go away, but taking ownership of your decision can help empower you, easing some of the pain. Encourage yourself with such positive assertions as, "As much as I want a child, I know I can't handle having one alone," or "I hope I find a man I want to marry because I desperately want a child, but I also desperately believe a child needs a father."

Even if you know for sure you do not want a child, you may be grieving your lost fantasies from childhood: playing house, pushing a doll carriage, choosing a name for your child. Don't be surprised by having a wave of sadness wash over you after you have come to a definitive decision. Don't be surprised if you go through this several times over a period of years. You are letting go of expectations and childhood dreams. Mourn their passing. The intensity of your grief will eventually abate.

If you decide to have a child, you may be proud of your decision, yet surprised—even during your excitement—at your occasional weepiness or outright grief. This may be a reaction to your major decision: you've defied societal rules that state a woman's life decisions revolve around a man. You've exerted your own wishes to shape your life. You may have done this despite the negative or skeptical reactions of family and friends. While being content with your decision, you may also be sad that you aren't having this child as part of a loving relationship. You may experience a full range of emotions.

Deciding to have a child without a husband can be both lonely and exciting. It may separate you from those people who are not as free as you to direct their own life. You may lose friends who are scared of such independent thinking. You may have unpleasant scenes with your family, who are afraid of being shamed by your decision (especially if you plan a pregnancy).

Even while being terribly excited about the surge of inner strength you feel from making this decision, and the upcoming changes in your life, you may—no, you *will*—have many moments of self-doubt. Be prepared. This is normal. Give the doubts room to exist; face your ambivalence. Let them teach you more about yourself. As you react to each doubt, you will feel more reassured of your decision. Don't overreact and don't panic; doubts will pass.

By answering all possible doubts or hesitations in advance, you will be reassured of the rightness of your decision. It is better to face your doubts and hesitations *before* your child arrives because, for certain, you—like all new mothers (even those with husbands)—will have doubts about your decision to have a child when your son or daughter cries inconsolably, or you've got to clean diapers and bedsheets at 3:00 AM.

If it's too late for you to consider being a mother, you may be nursing a low-grade sadness for the life you didn't have. This sadness is not pathological. It's perfectly normal to mourn the daughter or son you wanted.

In addition to grief, you may be angry at a particular man who rejected you or toward all men in general because, as Sally complained: "Men are so scared of commitment. They're the ones who prevent me from being a mother."

You may be angry at society for making a promise it couldn't keep: girls grow up to be wives and mothers. You may be angry that when you were of mothering age, it wasn't acceptable to adopt or have a child without a husband. You didn't have the opportunity to consider these options.

If possible, give yourself permission to feel the grief or anger; they often get entwined. Feel it. Talk about it. Dream about it. You will probably note that after a few weeks, the intensity of the feelings will subside and you will move, as one woman said, from "bitter to bittersweet." If your anger or bitterness doesn't abate, you may want to consult a therapist.

Self-Assessment

The third task, Making a Decision about Children, involves three key issues. Look them over to see how you are doing in each one.

Deciding If You Want To Have A Child

Deciding By Which Method You Want To Have A Child

Grieving Your Lost Dreams Of Motherhood—As Part Of A Marriage

For any category that you are satisfied with, give yourself a "star," either figuratively or literally. For any that you still need to work on, think about what needs to be added or changed in order for it to be satisfactory. Then, write your ideas for that category.

If you are stuck, talk with friends or family to see how they handle that task. If you are still stuck after that, consider reading a self-help book, taking a course that deals with the topic, or talking with a professional in the area, for example, your family physician or gynecologist, a fertility counselor, an adoption exchange organization, or a psychotherapist or religious counselor who specializes in single-parent families.

7

Enjoying Intimacy

"**M**y boss wanted to see me. I assumed it was about a promotion or at least a raise. I was flabbergasted when he fired me! I practically stumbled out of the office. I immediately drove home and called Doug. He said, 'I'm so sorry to hear that. Look, Eva, I'm busy now; it's not a good time to talk.'

"I could understand that, so I wasn't too upset. But what got me was he said he'd come by the next day after work. The next day! I had just been fired, and the next day was the best he could do!"

Eva's outrage spills forth as she recounts this story. "So I slammed down the phone and called my best friend, Patty. She said she'd have to rearrange an appointment for the afternoon, but she'd be over within a couple of hours. Now, that's a good friend; that's true intimacy!"

What Is Intimacy?

As a single woman, with or without a man, you need intimacy, the fourth task. In fact, without it, you may feel lonely, angry, or depressed. If you have a partner, like Eva, you may be lonely, angry, and/or depressed when he doesn't come through for you. If you don't have a partner, you may think that's the reason you are experiencing those feelings. While the absence of a lover may be one cause of loneliness or depression, the absence of intimacy is *always* a prime cause.

When you think of intimacy, what comes to mind? A quiet tête-à-tête with the man you love? Lying with him after lovemaking? Holding his hand as you walk through the woods or along the shore? Leaving work to be with your best friend who has just been fired? "Ah," you say, "that's different; that's not the same type of intimacy."

The Male Style Of Intimacy

Men *do* want intimacy; they want to be appreciated, valued, and loved. They want to feel special to a woman, and to hold her dear to their heart. However, research about intimacy among married and single men suggests this is an emotion they feel but can't define. When they do speak about it, they generally use the language of sex. Most men say they feel intimate with a woman when they are making love; some also add they feel intimate when lying together with her afterwards.

As a therapist, I hear married and single men talk about intimacy primarily in the context of problems in their relationships, rather than when things are going well. "We haven't been intimate [read, 'had sex'] for a long time," or "She doesn't like being intimate [read 'having sex'}."

For most men, lovemaking and emotional intimacy are synonymous. Sex is the language they use to express their need for emotional connection. Women often hear this as "just about sex." While for some men that may be true, the majority of men *do* want more emotional connection, but this is how they'll speak of it and show it. It's important you know the difference. (See Chapter 9 for more on men, intimacy, and sex.)

The Female Style Of Intimacy

For most women, lovemaking and emotional intimacy are *not* synonymous. Women value their style of intimacy, which includes personal sharing; they expect it from a man and are then disappointed when he can't provide it. That's why women need intimacy from women. Female friends have a special type of closeness to offer each other. In general, women tend to be more sensitive to emotions and more intuitive, so they can talk to each other in ways that men can't. This is poignantly portrayed by Terry McMillan in *Waiting to Exhale* (Pocket Books, 1992), which depicts the friendships among four middle class African-American women. What helps them through their problems with romances and careers is the power of their connection to each other.

There are times when a woman needs intimacy in her own style. In the example above, Doug most likely felt deep sympathy for Eva. When they got together the next day, he probably would be caring and supportive. Patty, on the other hand, dropped everything and came right over. Eva needed Patty's style of intimacy at that moment.

Whether or not you have a man in your life, you are more likely to have your emotional needs met by close female friends. If you don't have close female friends, you are likely to feel lonely, whether or not you have a man in your life.

If you are not aware of these differences, you may continue to seek emotional intimacy *solely* from a man, and then blame him (or the absence of a man) when you end up feeling unsatisfied or depressed.

Communication

You can't talk about intimacy for women without understanding the importance of communication. You can't talk about problems within male and female relationships without understanding the different ways men and women communicate. (See Chapter 9 for more on this subject.) Their different styles are well documented. In general, women show support through exploring and probing feelings. When a woman is upset about a situation, another woman will ask how she feels or will share a similar experience. Men, on the other hand, typically show support by being helpful and offering solutions. While men may feel sympathetic, their communication style differs so much from a woman's that she may feel put down, put off, or unsupported.

In *You Just Don't Understand* (Morrow, 1990), Deborah Tannen noted that in conversations, women "rapport" while men "report." This means that women want the rapport and personal connection that go along with the exchange of words. The connection, in fact, may be more important than the actual content of the discussion. When men talk, though, they report and exchange information. If they don't receive facts, they may feel dissatisfied with the conversation.

Neither style is better or worse than the other. Men may get the connection they want through talking with other men, just like women do in talking with other women. So, the problem comes when men and women are talking together. Unfortunately, though, too many single women blame themselves or blame men for not being able to be intimate, to talk with them in their female style.

My study supports what almost every other study on married and single women's friendship has found: women's emotional needs are better met by their close female friends, sisters, or mothers, than by their male friends or lovers.

Taking Friends For Granted

With women playing such a significant role in each other's emotional lives, it's important not to take female friendships for granted. Women don't take their love relationships for granted. Here, they spend time thinking how to make things better, how to please their lovers, and brooding over problems.

Why, then, do women devote so much more energy to nurturing a love relationship than an intimate friendship with another woman? Is this a pattern left over from high school, where female intimacy revolved around sharing secrets about boys? Where so little attention was paid to what happened between them as female friends? Is it a pattern left over from young adulthood, where friendships revolved around being comrades in the search for a man? Young women may have partied together, talked about boyfriend problems, and shared dreams of their ideal husband and wedding. The intimacy between them may always have taken second place to their sharing issues about males.

If a woman's close female friendships still revolve around men once she is past 30, they risk becoming too narrowly focused and stale. Emotionally neglecting your friendships—not nurturing them for their intimacy—may result in your reaching your 40s and 50s with a sense of emptiness, and then blaming that emptiness on the absence of a lover.

Eileen, a sociable woman in her early 40s, is a hostess in a restaurant. She is the type of woman who chats easily with others and is quick to make friends. As a long-time single, she has developed a large network of female friends and has a full social life. When talking about intimacy, she put into words what many women feel. "I'll always have my female friends, so I don't have to worry about that."

It doesn't occur to Eileen that she should worry a bit more about her close friends. Instead, she takes this attitude: "I don't expect as much from them as I do from men. I will put up with much more from a woman. If things get tense, I can just 'cool it' with her for a while and when we get back together in a few days, weeks, or even months, everything's forgotten."

Would she tolerate that from a man? "Absolutely *not!*"

To have a genuine sense of connection and intimacy, women—married and single—need to nurture the emotional intimacy they want within their female friendships. This accomplishes two things. First, it removes the pressure of finding that intense female-type intimacy with men. Without that requirement, you may be less dissatisfied with the men you are meeting. Second, you are more likely to maintain the closeness you have with women. Given the high rate of divorce and the frequency with which women change partners, men are more likely to move out of your life than your close female friends.

Pruning The Friendship Garden

I was amazed to learn from my study how many women have close friends (as distinguished from social or convenience friends, or just acquaintances) going back to college days, high school, and, yes, even elementary school. Always Single and Single Again women have close friends they've known for 25 or more years. Yet, being in such a mobile society, women rarely continue to live near their close friends.

Women tend to hold on to their old close friends while making few new ones. It is especially difficult for women who move to a new city to establish new friendships. They may not reach out to other women, and women who have their own friendship network may not reach out to a newcomer. The data on friendships also suggest that out of loyalty to their old friendships, women may not take the opportunity to choose different types of new friends, reflecting the personal growth they've made over the years.

To make sure your old close friendships grow with you as you grow and change, take a critical look at them. Do you invest the time and energy in them that you do for your career or your relationship with a lover? Or do you take them for granted like children do their parents: not showing or expressing your love and affection, assuming they'll always be there; not assuming they can evolve along with your own growth in maturity?

Few women would treat problems in a love relationship with the same non-chalance Eileen does with her friends. With lovers, if there are difficulties, women tend to call, write, or talk with the man—over and over again—trying to solve the problems. And if the relationship must end, women devote a lot of energy to understanding what went wrong.

When there is a problem with your close female friends, do you, like Eileen, ignore it, assuming the friendship will always be there? Or, do you challenge each other by confronting the problems? If you face the issues together, you both may grow and change. In reality, though, many long-term friendships become awkward or dissatisfying. So, women avoid facing the problem head on and just drift apart.

Typically, whether because of the stress or the dissatisfaction, one or the other friend stops calling or stops returning the other's calls. Unfortunately, too often it doesn't even occur to women to think about friendship as something that needs to be maintained.

When there isn't a man in your life, close friends become even more important since they may be your only source of true nurturance and intimacy. Therefore, when you maintain unpruned and outgrown friendships, you may be depriving yourself of necessary nutrients, whether you have or don't have a man. As with plants, the lack of nutrients may lead to a stunting of your emotional, personal, and perhaps even your professional growth.

Two years ago, Marsha's depression caused her to take a temporary leave of absence from the airline where she had worked for many years. A single mother of four adolescents, she felt she was drowning in everyone else's needs— her children's, her friends', her colleagues'. She was always there for others, but friends rarely came through for her, even after her suicide attempt.

One day I asked Marsha to draw a picture, representing her current friendships through the metaphor of a garden. She started slowly with a few marks on the paper, then as the idea of the garden took hold, the crayons began whipping around the page. She drew an overcast day with a circle of muted colored flowers and weeds.

As she looked at her completed picture, I asked, "Do the weeds need to be pulled or just transplanted to the border?"

She thought for a second, then said, "That would leave room for me to find new friends in the center, wouldn't it?"

"Would you like to draw a picture showing how you would *like* your friendship garden to look?"

Marsha picked up the crayons. A few minutes later she sat back and reflected on the two pictures. "The first one is less clear, the colors aren't as bright; there's no sun. In the center the flowers are drowned out by the weeds. In the second one, there are birds and a sun. The faded flowers are still there, but many of them are moved to the edges with room left in the middle for new ones. The weeds have been moved to outside the fence. And, everything is brighter and clearer."

Marsha could see by doing this exercise how she had settled for more weeds in her life than she wanted, which led to her feeling lonely and starved for intimacy. She keeps some of her friends, represented as "faded flowers," in the center of her garden. In order to make them brighter, she must learn to ask for what she needs and to confront difficulties that arise with her friends. With the extra space in the middle of the garden, she has room for new friends in her life. That, of course, means learning to choose new friends who can give back to her. (For an excellent resource on women's friendships, see *Among Friends* by Letty Cottin Pogrebin [McGraw-Hill, 1987].)

Evolving Friendships

If you are to rely on your female friends for the intimacy that will keep you feeling connected and content, you need to be sure, unlike Eileen and Marsha, that your friends continue to reflect who you are as you develop. If they remain static, however, you may realize you are outgrowing them. Many women, though, reject the concept of "outgrowing" friends.

As you physically grow and mature, you outgrow some of your old clothes; items you used to like no longer fit nor reflect who you have become. So, why don't we consider outgrowing friends? Think about friendships as evolving. When you and your friends grow and evolve in different directions, when you no longer have similar interests and ideas about intimacy, perhaps you need to retire some of them—if not from your life entirely, then from the center of your garden.

What you needed from your 20-year-old college roommate is probably not what you need from your 43- or 65-year-old best friend today. Let me tell you an experience from my own life.

As college roommates, Robyne and I were extreme opposites, but despite our differences, we were best friends. For the first eight years of our friendship, we helped each other learn about the adult world, about men, and about ourselves.

A decade later, though, Robyne was in a traditional marriage and I was advancing professionally as a therapist. While these differences can work for some friends, we felt deprived because we couldn't get from each other what we wanted. We each blamed the other for not giving enough; we slowly pulled away, recognizing we had outgrown our original friendship. Some friends can grow together; we hadn't. We knew we eventually had to say goodbye to the specialness that we had shared in our early adulthood.

We decided to meet and talk about our changed expectations for our friendship. Over egg rolls and moo shi chicken, we reminisced about how important those early years had been for us. We laughed over our old fights, like when she poured ketchup over my head—or had I done it to her? Although it was awkward, we talked about needing to redefine our friendship. We knew we wanted to keep in touch somehow, maybe just a yearly update. Robyne is still in my friendship garden, but she is planted at the outer edges.

Robyne and I both recognized we were growing apart. While always painful, the growing apart is even more difficult when only one of the friends is dissatisfied. As that one pulls away, the other one feels rejected. Neither woman may really understand what is happening.

Pat and Lynn are in their early 50s. They had been friends since high school. After graduation, both took jobs in the same office of a large personnel company. Over the years, Pat moved up in management, while Lynn was satisfied with her middle-level supervisory position.

The two women did not understand that their relationship was changing. They had spent many hours in their 20s, 30s, and 40s talking about men, joining tennis and ski clubs, taking Club Med vacations together. A major theme for their friendship was their mutual survival as singles in a world that values marriage.

When Pat became depressed, she entered therapy. As she began making changes in her life, she noticed she was less depressed—except when she was with Lynn. She realized that a hallmark of their friendship had been griping about how bad things were with men, with their family, at the office.

As Pat became more assertive with her family and at work, and expanded her interests, she was less interested in moaning about men. While she still wanted to meet a man, she was not *actively* looking. This put a wedge between Lynn and her.

Lynn, for her part, felt deserted by this "new" Pat. The more Pat pulled away, the more Lynn attempted to draw closer, which Pat experienced as clinging, which caused her to pull still further away. The tension between them rose. Pat eventually slithered away from the friendship by changing jobs. Lynn never understood what happened and was left with a bucket full of unresolved feelings.

Books, movies, songs all recount the pain of falling out of love. How many stories or songs do you know, though, about the pain of falling out of close friendships? Sometimes, the hurt of losing a friend can be even deeper than losing a lover. You may fear you won't meet another woman who can be such a good friend. You certainly won't meet another woman who is part of your history! Pat later realized she had been willing to put up with a less-than-satisfying friendship with Lynn because, "The devil you know is better than the one you don't." They had shared so much together; she wasn't sure she'd ever find another friend with whom she could feel the same closeness she had with Lynn.

Unfortunately, Pat and Lynn lost an opportunity to hold on to the memories of their closeness while mourning together the loss of their current friendship.

Without this joint grieving (the same as with ex-lovers), it may be hard to be emotionally open to new friends.

Toxic Friends

Pat and Lynn started out with a genuine friendship that met the needs of both women. Over the decades, however, it evolved into what Florence Isaacs calls a "toxic friendship." In *Toxic Friends, True Friends* (Morrow, 1999), she describes toxic friendships as those that *regularly* are unsupportive, unrewarding, unsatisfying, draining, and stifling.

Think about your friendships in this context. Do you have close friends who are mean to you? Who leave you feeling less than good about yourself? Maybe the friendship started with one of you being more needy or more dependent than the other, but over time there has been a shift. Now, you are uncomfortable with that imbalance. Rules for friendships, as we saw with Pat and Lynn, can change. The outcome can be a lack of respect for one another or a feeling of being stifled.

Toxic friendships can also result from unrealistic expectations; when one woman rushes a friendship; when there is an unhealthy envy or competitiveness; or when conflict is ignored. All of these situations coat a close friendship with distrust and disillusionment, which means that your intimacy needs are not being met by these friends.

Differences In Female-Style Intimacy

Intimacy means different things to different women. What one woman thinks is intimate, another thinks is smothering, and a third thinks is just being sociable. Our degree of comfort with intimacy comes from our cultural or ethnic styles, through absorbing our family's (sometimes unspoken) rules about closeness, and through recognizing the different levels of closeness compatibility. If you understand this, you can recognize and appreciate that differences between friends may be more a matter of style than a barrier to intimacy.

Cultural And Ethnic Styles Of Closeness

While we should be cautious about stereotyping people, some cultural and ethnic patterns do shape the way people express their intimacy. This has been well documented by a number of books on ethnicity, most notably *Ethnicity and Family Therapy*, edited by family therapists Monica McGoldrick, John Pearce, and Joseph Giordano (Guilford, 1997).

Certainly, these cultural influences will be affected by the number of generations a family has lived in the United States. Also, most people have parents from two different cultural backgrounds, so there may be more influence from one side or the other. These ideas need to be put into perspective, however; and knowing these differences can sometimes prevent misunderstandings.

For example, women of African-American, Italian, Jewish, and Mediterranean heritages often relate in a more emotionally open style than women of British, German, Asian, and Scandinavian descent. The former tend to be freer with touch, verbal affection, and compliments. The latter may be more reserved with their comments and stand slightly further apart when talking to others.

Rachel and Anna, long-time friends and coworkers, are driving Maria, a new employee, home. While Anna sits quietly in the back, Rachel and Maria talk about how difficult it is being single in a small southern town.

Maria, of Puerto Rican heritage, confides in them: "I've only been here a few months, but I'm worried about being lonely. In Chicago, it was no big deal. I had lots of single friends and the city is really set up for us. How do I meet men if there are no places for singles to hang out?"

Rachel, a Jewish woman from New York, smiles. "I'm sorry to report, but it's true; being single here *is* hard. There are only a few places where women go by themselves, without its being a meat market."

The conversation soon drifts off to other topics, including Maria and Rachel sharing their thoughts about adopting a child. When Maria is dropped off, Anna moves to the front seat and instantly proclaims, "I don't like her." Surprised, Rachel asks why. "She shared too much personal stuff—being lonely, meeting men, adopting a baby." Anna shudders, "She hardly knows us!"

For Anna, a fourth-generation German on both sides, it takes lots of time and frequent contact to build such familiarity. Anna is a lively person who talks freely with others, but about things and ideas, not personal feelings. She must know someone a long time before she will do that. To her, what Rachel and Maria had shared was intensely private. To them, they were just being sociable, sympathetic, and helpful.

The Family's Rules Of Closeness

Along with their cultural or ethnic styles, most families have their own rules of intimacy. Sometimes these rules are homegrown homilies, such as "Friends come and go but your family is always there." "Blood is thicker than water." "You're stuck with your family, but you choose your friends." These rules are rarely written, and sometimes not even spoken, but children learn their family's rules by observing how their parents relate to others.

Whether you adore your family or refuse to see them, you still honor their rules. Interestingly, the more conflictual your relationship with your parents, the more likely you are to live by their codes! (For more on dealing with family rules, see Chapter 11.)

The Thompsons have been a Midwestern farming family for three generations. The children were expected to come straight home from school to do their farm chores. Friends weren't for socializing; they were for crises, such as after a windstorm when extra hands were needed to patch the barn quickly before the coming rains.

After the two oldest Thompson children graduated from the community college, they chose to remain on the farm. Jessica, the youngest, moved to New York to study dancing when she came of age. Her parents and siblings refused to have anything to do with a child who would "desert" them.

For the next ten years Jessica had minimal contact with her family. But something was seriously wrong with her life. When she began therapy, she was not dancing to her potential, was having frequent accidents that required emergency attention, and although she had many acquaintances, had no close friends.

As she talks about her loneliness, Jessica realizes how much she has honored the family code. "Oh, goodness; it's so clear now. 'Friends are for emergencies only,' so I can feel close to friends only through my accidents!"

She talks about how she always felt torn between her desire to dance and her sense of obligation to help her father on the farm. "I thought by coming East, I had left all that behind. But I guess I'm still stuck with the same dilemma. Do I really get down to serious dancing or not? If I do, how do I deal with the feeling of turning my back on them?"

This is an important question. If she chooses to stay in New York, she will have to deal with her family more directly. She'll have to find a way to resolve rejecting their way of life, but not *them,* and choosing a career that satisfies who she is. She must find a way to value their way of life—for them—while still valuing her own. She needs to genuinely acknowledge, by letter or in person, how she has hurt them by abandoning their lifestyle. She needs to express an interest in what is happening at home, as well as telling them about her dancing and her daily life—even if they don't seem interested. She needs to think about what she gained from her farm life and her family life that gives her the strength to take on the challenge of moving to a new environment with no supports.

If she can do this, Jessica can free herself from guilt. Only then will she be emotionally free to change those family rules that no longer work for her. She will be able to have friends because she likes them, not needs them. She can get serious about her dancing. Then she can stay on the East Coast and dance while still feeling connected to her family. If she does this, then their acceptance of her decisions, while it would be nice, is not necessary for her to feel settled and emotionally free to establish her own life and to develop close friends.

Different Levels Of Closeness Compatibility

Not recognizing that people have different levels of closeness compatibility—whether because of cultural or family rules—can interfere with one's ability to find intimacy. Without this awareness, women may personalize problems in their friendships or blame the other woman for not caring enough.

Think about the type of women you have been, or wanted to be, friendly with over the years. Were there some who smothered you, calling too often, offering to do too much for you? Were there some that you knew liked you, yet they seemed so aloof, as if they were sending you a double message about being friends? If you think about closeness as a continuum from one to ten, with one being more reserved and ten being more emotionally open, you'll recognize that you would place some of your friends at the lower end of the scale and assign others the higher numbers.

We can see how this works with Anna and Rachel. It took a few years for Anna to feel comfortable with Rachel. In the beginning, Rachel felt betrayed that Anna never shared her feelings. Rachel, one of four sisters from a Jewish family, places herself on the upward end of the closeness compatibility scale, at a 7 or 8. Anna, an only child, describes herself as a 2 or 3. No wonder Rachel felt that Anna was "withholding" from her.

Rather than personalizing the strain in their friendship, and thus blaming either herself or Anna, Rachel learned to see that their differences were just a matter of style. She adjusted her expectations for the friendship and backed off for almost a year. Anna, on the other hand, experienced Rachel as intrusive, so when Rachel backed off from the friendship, it felt totally appropriate, allowing Anna to move slowly toward their getting to know each other better.

Reflection: Compatibility Scale

To see how the compatibility level scale fits for you, think about a number that represents a comfortable degree of closeness. Now, try assigning numbers to your close friends. Do you notice any patterns? Are all your close friends within a few numbers of you? Do you see why some of your friendships flow smoother than others?

Now think about women you wanted to know better who ignored you or pushed you away. Think about women who tried to become close with you, whom you ignored or pushed away. Give them numbers and see how close you were on the scale.

Sometimes it works better having close friends with similar numbers, but as we saw with Anna and Rachel, sometimes—if you are patient—it is worth waiting for your timing to come into sync.

Rules For Your Friendships

Keeping in mind cultural style, family rules, and compatibility differences, still other general issues apply to all close friendships. Drawing from Isaacs's *Toxic Friends, True Friends,* here is a list of what she calls "Rules for Friendship."

- be direct
- express your feelings without attacking
- listen carefully and empathize with your friend

- communicate early when you have concerns
- don't ignore the problem, letting it fester
- be aware of sensitive issues
- don't betray a confidence
- don't fail to reciprocate
- make an effort to get together
- celebrate a friend's success

As you probably noticed, this could also be a list for having a healthy love relationship. Intimacy, whether with a man or a woman, romantic or platonic, calls for the same emotional investment, and the same attention to these friendship rules.

Making New Friends After 35

When you were younger, you were more likely to "fall into friendship" like people "fall in love." You'd meet a girl and become fast friends. After college, though, the daily opportunities to meet others usually decrease. You go from being thrown together to having to seek out women, to choose whom you want for friends. Now, you're more likely to "slide into friendship" by first making the acquaintance of colleagues, neighbors, day care mothers, committee members. Some of these people may become convenience or activity friends and only over time, if ever, become close friends.

What makes it even harder to make new friends in midlife is that women who are settled with their friendship network are not necessarily open to making new friends. Rita was married for 12 years. During those years, she had developed many close friends—first through her children's day care, then later through their sports and dance programs. When her husband left her, she returned to college, then got a job in retail. After so many years in the same area, she has good friends from different parts of her life.

Rachel met Rita at a business meeting. They appeared to like each other, but whenever Rachel suggested they get together, Rita never had time. At first Rachel assumed that meant Rita didn't like her, yet when they talked, it seemed she did. After her experience with her coworker Anna, Rachel was more sensitive to cultural differences. But this didn't seem related to that. Rachel was angry that she was getting mixed messages from Rita.

Contrary to what happened between Pat and Lynn, Rachel confronted Rita. She was surprised to hear: "Of course I like you. I like you a lot, but my dance card is full. I just don't have time to think about calling anyone else. I barely have time for the friends I already have."

Rachel was annoyed at Rita's response, but at least she understood and didn't need to personalize it: "Rita's not wanting to be with me because she doesn't like me." Rachel can choose to persist in initiating contact with Rita, and maybe over time they will become closer. Or Rachel can accept Rita as a woman she likes but will probably never get to know better.

Don't Confuse The Absence Of Intimacy With The Absence Of A Man

If you are without close friends, or if you have problems with your close friendships, you may feel a general dissatisfaction with life. Not recognizing that that dissatisfaction comes from the loss of female intimacy, you may blame it on the lack of a man. Some women, not understanding that, make matters worse by spending more time and creativity looking for a man than improving a friendship or looking for female friends. You may miss having a man in your life, and this could, of course, leave you feeling lonely. But the intensity of your feelings may be related more to the absence or loss of close friends than to the lack of a man.

While finding both a man and a close female friend are difficult, you actually have more opportunity to meet women who might evolve into close friends and who can meet your intimacy needs than you do to find a man who is emotionally available for a relationship. Therefore, you might consider putting more effort into improving your female friendships or meeting new women so that you will feel less lonely when there is no man in your life.

Self-Assessment

The fourth task, Enjoying Intimacy, involves four key issues. Look them over to see how you are doing in each one.

Defining Intimacy

___don't take your friends for granted

Pruning Your Friendship Garden

___assess the quality of your friendships
___question if you have outgrown any of your friends
___consider if you need different types of friends to fit who you are today
___assess if you have any toxic friends

Understanding Differences In Friendship Styles

___identify cultural differences
___identify family rules about closeness
___identify different levels of closeness

Making New Friends

___recognize the difficulty of doing this

For any category that you are satisfied with, give yourself a "star," either figuratively or literally. For any that you still need to work on, think about what needs to be added or changed in order for it to be satisfactory. Then, write your ideas for that category.

If you are stuck, talk with friends or family to see how they handle that task. If you are still stuck after that, consider reading a self-help book, taking a course on women's friendships, or talking with a professional counselor or religious leader.

Hope For Horniness—Facing Your Sexual Feelings

The fifth task is to take control of your sexual feelings when you don't have a partner. Although society is more open to sexually explicit conversations than ever before, people are still reluctant to talk about a woman's horniness.

The Itch: Sexuality Is A Core Part Of Being A Woman

When you don't have a partner, what do you do with your sensual, feminine, sexy feelings? With your sexual feelings that erupt at their own whim, not asking your permission, and arising at the most inopportune times?

For example, you are premenstrual and sitting in a business meeting. You suddenly become acutely, sensually aware of a man's leg brushing up against yours. You are putting lotion on your legs and feel a rippling sensation throughout your body. Watching an exotic sunset or staying overnight in a hotel, you feel sexually passionate. Even something as ordinary as walking down the street can become erotic as you feel the sensual movement of your body. And sometimes, for no reason at all, you just feel horny.

Being aware of these sensual feelings may be wonderful, but at times sensual feelings remind you of what you don't have—sexual fulfillment within a loving relationship.

Some midlife women, actively hoping to meet a man, may acknowledge these sensations, keeping their sensuality available and ready against the time when, who knows, they may run into "him" in the grocery store, on a bus, or just walking down the street.

For other midlife women, however, years of unfulfilled hope in finding a partner have them spending less psychic energy thinking about meeting a man and, consequently, little need for a readied sensuality. For them, knowing they can awaken their sexuality (even if it takes a bit more time) is sufficient. They prefer not to have a heightened sensuality be an active part of their life.

The fact is, though, you don't have a choice about the arrival of these feelings. They have a mind of their own. You can tell yourself you aren't interested in men, but it's not as easy to tell your body to stop having sexual feelings.

In a therapy session, Joanna (who we'll meet in Chapter 9) shares excerpts from her journal.

"I touch my cheek; it is so soft. It's hard to believe there may never be anyone else touching it. The softness makes me feel so sensuous, not really sexy, but 'lovely.' I must be careful; allowing myself to feel that is dangerous; it makes me too depressed.

"I think I have accepted the possibility that I will never be with another man. But then these feelings well up, and I can't believe I'll be alone forever. I try to imagine myself at 50 without a man. If I work hard at it, I can actually imagine it without seeing me depressed and miserable. That is, until I touch my cheek again. The only solution is to not feel my soft cheek, to shut down the part of me that enjoys feeling so lovely."

Joanna felt "shutting down" was her only option. She didn't know she had at least three options for dealing with her sexual feelings.

Think about sexual feelings as an itch; they are a normal bodily sensation. *Acknowledgment,* option one, means being aware of the itch and scratching it. But what if you can't scratch the itch? You might need to go through any number of contortions for relief, or you might learn to ignore the itch by distracting yourself. This is the second option, *distraction.* The third option, *denial,* is training yourself not to feel the itch in the first place. This is what Joanna referred to as shutting down.

With acknowledgment, you're aware when you feel horny, when you're aroused. You may tend to those feelings (that is, masturbate, fantasize, have sex), or you may sit them out, knowing they're there, but not doing anything. You just let them pass. The potential hazard in full acknowledgment is freneticism, obsessively thinking about and looking for a man.

With distraction, you make a conscious effort to distract yourself from feeling horny, not just for the moment, but in general. You know the sexual energy and passion are there, but you turn them in another direction, toward work or a volunteer project or a hobby. With distraction, you can access the feeling when you want to by consciously turning that energy back to your body.

You may find that you move back and forth between acknowledgment and distraction. For example, in acknowledgment, you may enjoy expressing your sensuality in your dress or body language. But you may temporarily choose to distract some of that energy when in a business meeting. On the other hand, even if you distract your sexual energy, there may be times you choose to access those sexual feelings, like when you just meet an interesting man. If that relationship ends, you have the choice to return to distraction or to remain in acknowledgment.

Unlike distraction, denial is an unconscious process. Here, you have de-pressed your feelings so deeply that you cannot feel them. By numbing your sexual energy, you may experience an emotional flatness. The potential hazard of long-term denial may be depression or a deadened personality.

Physiologically, postmenopausal women may be harder to arouse, and so they may not be able to choose full-time acknowledgment.

If this sounds mechanical, it is. But the reality is that you already are making the choice among these options, only you do it unconsciously, without any control about your choice. This way, you make a conscious choice, and you maintain a sense of control—not over *having* the horny feelings, but what to do with them.

Acknowledging The Itch

It is easy to acknowledge your sexual feelings when you are involved with a man. However, if you choose to be open to these feelings when there is no man in your life, you must decide how to deal with them. When acknowledging the feelings, many women turn to self-destructive behaviors just to be able to scratch the itch. Combine this with society's pressure for you to be partnered, and you may end up frantically looking for men or getting involved with inappropriate ones.

Your first choice for dealing with your sexual feelings may be having a loving partner. When that's not an option, however, you'll want to consider other means for sexual release.

Masturbation

Shirley says people describe her as "mousy." Today, she looks it, sitting in my office wearing a gray, shapeless dress. In her soft voice, she tells me about a recent conversation with Judith, her best friend, who has been married for nine years.

"I was talking about feeling horny. I said, 'I bet you can't imagine how awful it is not to have had sex for three years!' And, would you believe, Judith said, 'You can always masturbate.' I know she was only trying to be helpful, but really. . . ."

At this, Shirley stops talking and shrinks even further into the chair. But suddenly her face turns red as she screams, "Even my best friend can't understand!"

Most single women who are not in a sexual relationship *can* understand Shirley's dilemma. No matter how inventive you are, masturbation is not the same as sex with a loving partner. For some women, the physiological release is less important than the physical and emotional touching that comes from sex with a loving partner.

Shirley may look mousy, but she speaks in colorful images. "Sometimes masturbating is like a mechanical sexual release, something you do regularly, like a car tune-up. Periodically, I make sure it's still working because my gynecologist said, 'Use it or lose it.' I thought that was rather tacky of him; it's not like I have a lot of choices. So, like with a tune-up, I masturbate to make sure my oils still flow. I may 'come,' though, with huge sobs, sobs of loneliness. No, it's more than that. I'm resentful that I have no choice."

Some women have an entirely different experience from Shirley's. They find masturbation very sensual; they make it an event. They might lower the lights or burn incense. They might listen to romantic or soothing music. In choosing the setting, they may soak in a bubble bath with candles around the tub, lie on their bed watching erotic videos and using a vibrator, model sexy clothing in front of their mirror.

While some women create elaborate sexual fantasies as they masturbate, others use boring and repetitive ones. If you need new ideas, you may want to read *My Secret Garden* (Pocketbooks, 1973). Nancy Friday collected sexual fantasies from women of all ages. Although published nearly three decades ago, it is still a valuable bedside companion.

For some women, getting aroused takes too much effort. They may have no particular desire to masturbate. But, like Shirley, they need to check that the oil still flows. For them, masturbation is not erotic; it is purely a physiological release. There's no fantasizing, no enjoyment, but neither is there a sense of loneliness.

Shirley describes how she wishes she could experience masturbation. "You're hungry, you eat. You're thirsty, you drink. You're horny or tense, you masturbate. Sometimes you make a feast of the meal, and sometimes you just eat or drink to satisfy your physical need."

Male Friend

Some women have a male friend whom they see primarily for sex. This seldom is a relationship of great emotional satisfaction, but it provides companionship and is one in which a woman can have her sexual and tactile needs met. In this arrangement, the man and woman may see each other regularly, but have sex only when one or the other is feeling horny. Or, they may see each other strictly when they want to have sex.

If you don't fall into the trap of making more out of the relationship than you know it can support, this can be a satisfactory option. The main thing is to be honest about your expectations and to protect yourself from feeling let down by his not having more to offer you.

Polygamy

Years ago, Elena Lessner, a fellow therapist from New York, wrote an unpublished spoof about polygamy, addressing the numerical problem of more available single women than single men. In countries that support polygamy, the women are at the mercy of the man's power and control. However, as Lessner describes it, polygamy can benefit the women as much as the man, if they don't give up their personal power. Since a man is often attracted to similar types, the women might like each other and become good friends. They may or may not become lovers themselves.

The advantages for the man are obvious: more women to meet his needs.

But there are also advantages for the women. They get to have a relationship with a man and a close friendship with a woman—who can offer the type of emotional intimacy they probably can't have with him. Plus, by living together and sharing expenses, a polygamous threesome would have a definite financial advantage. Looked at in this light, the arrangement doesn't seem so farfetched.

However, some women might have moral and/or emotional problems with polygamy. Morally, they may be opposed on sexual grounds. Emotionally, they may not like knowing the man they love is making love to another woman, even with prior agreement.

Affairs With Married Men

Let's face it. Polygamy won't be taken seriously by singles, but a solution that many women do choose is similar to polygamy, with the main difference being the secrecy and lack of power: namely, having an affair. While statistics are impossible to establish, estimates run as high as one out of every two women having been in an affair with a married man.

For years, the "other woman" has been seen as self-destructive, pathetic, or a siren. Yet, I've seen significant changes in my practice over the past three decades. Women are choosing to have affairs, aware of the limitations, yet finding some satisfaction in this arrangement. These are not pathetic or helpless women. This suggests that despite stereotypes, women can be emotionally healthy and have an affair. They may choose a man who's in a stale marriage who uses the affair to learn new ways of giving and receiving. The women can set higher expectations for his emotional involvement because they have less to lose if he refuses.

Rosie is an Always Single 44-year-old artist. Because of her age, she has reluctantly given up her wish to have children, but she refuses to give up her wish to be married. However, until she meets an appropriate man, she does not want to rule out being loved and having sex.

She is telling a group of women about her affairs. "I bring out the best in men. Because I don't need a married man, if he wants to be with me, he must be more attentive to me and my feelings. I only want an honest relationship, with clean fighting. And, the good news is that some married men, far more than single men, are willing to try harder to work out problems rather than just leave."

Interestingly, women in my study felt the gains from their affairs far outweighed any of the pains. Most often, they talked about gaining a good friend. They had a man who loved and cared for them, plus their sexual needs were being satisfied. A number of women said knowing that they could love and care for a man raised their self-confidence. They loved the romance and the fullness of being loved that the affair gave to their lives. Some women admitted that the affairs took the pressure off them to heed that old message: find a man.

"The bad news about affairs," Rosie adds, "is that as the man learns how to relate more emotionally, he goes back to use the new skills with his wife." She gives a bitter laugh. "I console myself, though, with knowing how many marriages I have helped!"

If you are having an affair, or you are considering one, here are some ideas for taking control of the situation so you can protect yourself. Heeding the cautions of women who have had affairs may help you take the good from the relationship and avoid the harm.

First and foremost, you need to find a way to organize the affair so you won't feel resentful that you are just part of the man's life and that your time together must revolve around his wife and children.

Second, you need to accept that only some of your needs are going to be met; you must protect yourself from feeling "one down" or "poor me" in competition with his wife. You need to protect yourself from believing his proclamation that his wife is to blame for their marital problems. Most important, you need to protect yourself from not expecting more from a married man than he can give—despite his persistent promises to divorce his wife and marry you.

Third, be cautious of what my friend Emily Brown, in *Affairs: A Guide to Working through the Repercussions of Infidelity* (Jossey Bass, 1999), calls "exit affairs." This is where a man uses the affair to ready himself to leave his wife—but not necessarily to take up with you!

One way to protect yourself is to establish some boundaries. For instance, see him as an *addition* to your already full life, not counting on him to fill your life. You are less likely to feel angry and used if you fit him into *your* schedule, rather than you fitting into his.

Another form of boundary setting is to limit and formalize the contact. Some women find an ongoing relationship with a married man too emotionally painful. They feel safe only with a "same time next year" (or next month) affair. This way, they can use their time between encounters to get on with their life and still have a designated time—outside of their daily routine—to be sensual and feel loved. I hear from numerous women that yearly professional conferences become "an island outside of real life" for an ongoing love affair.

At some point, many women decide what they are getting from a married man may not be worth the price they are paying, or they feel bad about deceiving another woman. Then they end the affair. But remember, as an old professor of mine once said, "Any damn fool can have an affair; it takes real skill to end one." In the best of all possibilities, the enjoyment of the affair is yours and the decision to move on is yours too.

Women With Women

Loving another woman is an option that's gaining wider social acceptance. Some women have turned to other women for their emotional and sexual needs and discovered a comfort they had not experienced with men. Some come to recognize they are lesbians who have denied that part of their identity.

Other women see a female relationship as temporary, filling the gap until they meet a man. They ask, "Why should I deprive myself of physical and emotional intimacy just because I've not met a sensitive, caring man who is not afraid of intimacy?"

Still other women become aware of their bisexuality. They feel sexually attracted to men and women. While it's more socially acceptable to be with a man, bisexual women may feel that working on a mutually healthy relationship with a man takes too much effort and gives too few rewards. Some feel their needs are better understood by another woman, and being with one is easier and offers more emotional satisfaction.

A young female client recently was telling me about her heterosexual relationships, but wondered if she were really bisexual. She had hated the thought of not being "normal," until she heard a reassuring lecture. The speaker said: "Bisexuals really are the luckiest people of all. They can choose their partners based solely on the person, not on the genitals."

If the social stigma of being lesbian or bisexual were removed, women could be free to experiment with all aspects of their sexuality and find what best fits them. It may be that their emotional needs are better met by another woman. It also may be that while enjoying the lesbian relationship, they acknowledge their primary sexual attraction is toward men.

Distracting The Itch

"One of the many parts I love about being menopausal is not having sexual feelings. They aren't jumping up and biting me all the time. They aren't making me horny; they aren't making me feel depressed that I'm not getting sex." Lots of women make similar comments. It's a relief not to have to deal with sexual feelings if you aren't in a relationship.

But for women whose bodies are still sexually vibrant, they do have to deal with the feelings when there's no outlet with a consenting adult. If you rule out full-time acknowledgment, then one way to distract yourself from your sex drive is to redirect the energy away from your body. You may pursue other sensuous activities—such as working with pottery or gardening or dancing. You may find a type of outreach that fulfills your own needs to give and receive, such as tutoring children who need your affection, or volunteering at an animal shelter. Or you may turn to your work, not as an avoidance of men—as some people claim—but because you have more unused energy.

Many single women who are not involved with a man and are using distraction talk about feeling "more centered" than when they are in a relationship or actively looking for a man. That may be because in redirecting your sexual feelings, the energy goes into something else that adds to your sense of fulfillment and competence.

"My life is fuller now," says Bonnie, after she ended an unsatisfying relationship of a few months. "I am spending more time with my girlfriends; I'm going back to doing the things I let go when I was dating Louis. I hate to admit it, but I really do feel better about myself when I'm not dating and not out there looking.

"Well, let me be a bit more honest. There are still moments I feel real sad, but they don't last so long, and they just come each month before my period. So I cry myself to sleep, and the next day, I'm back to feeling good within myself."

Yes, crying is a good distraction from pressing sexual needs, whether they are from deep longing or from a physiological basis. If this fits for you, give yourself permission to cry. You may even make it a lovely experience. Arrange a soothing and nurturing setting, and then let the tears—and the sobs—run free. Bonnie adds, "I usually hate when it starts, but afterwards, it's wonderful; it's like a 'come,' a sexual release. Then I get back to where I was before—comfortable with my life without the sexual pressure."

Denying The Itch

The major difference between denial and distraction is that redirecting your feelings is a conscious attempt to remove the sexual feelings. Removing them still leaves you with your vibrant juices that can be transferred to other areas of your life and reactivated when you choose. Denying or numbing the feeling is the process of making it disappear.

Contrary to the popular image, many single women go years without having a sexual relationship. After pursuing numerous unsuccessful pathways to finding a man, some believe the best way to cope with arousal is to deaden the feeling. These women no longer feel the desire. The longer they go without sex, the easier it is to numb their sexual, sensual feelings.

Ruth is a quiet, thoughtful woman. Now 57, her husband died when she was 38. While she has dated a bit, she found it more distasteful to be with men who can't really talk with her than to be alone. "After so many years," she says, "you get used to no one touching you. After a while, you stop thinking about it. How? It just happens. Your mind gets set to the point that it doesn't bother you, and it doesn't. I don't think about sex any more."

Ruth is quite attractive, but she wears an expression that says "I'm tired of trying and failing." She shifts in the chair and drops her voice as she confesses: "I'll tell you something. If I'm watching TV and there's a love scene, I have to turn my head. I guess it bothers me to see something like that. You get used to numbing it out, and watching it stirs up the feelings again, so you have to keep them pushed away."

If you are too successful in numbing your sexual feelings, you may not be able to reactivate them when you want. Not only can you become "dried out" sexually, other parts of your life may also become emotionally hardened because of your lack of sexual energy. Danny (married) and Linda (Always Single) were good friends and colleagues. One day Danny asked: "What's different about you? You seem . . . I don't know the word, but almost softer." Linda blushed, but had no answer.

Later that night, she recalled his comment and immediately thought about the prior weekend. She had spent it with a man, and had had sex for the first time in more than four years. Her partner had been nice, but nothing special. At first Linda dismissed any connection between her encounter and Danny's observation, but as she later reported: "I think I blushed because I *did* feel different. Maybe softer is the right word. I wasn't aware how I'd tightened up against those [sexual] feelings, but it was as if something inside had sort of melted."

Another potential problem with successful numbing is that you might exert so much energy containing the feelings, for fear they will slip out, that you become more rigid and less playful. Pejorative terms like "spinster" and "old maid" might have originated from society observing women who had deadened their sensual feelings beyond a retrievable point.

Finally, growing numb to your feelings can be hazardous to your physical health. If you are numb for too long, your body may react physiologically. Problems such as eczema, acne, diarrhea, stomach cramps, and headaches may occur as a result of shutting down your feelings.

Joanna wrote in her journal that the only solution to her horniness was to shut down her sexual feelings. If she thought about these three options—acknowledgment, distraction, and denial—she still might not like her choices, but at least she could take control and make the choice. She still might decide to shut down her feelings, or she might think about ways to distract herself at these moments, or she might allow herself the sensuousness of touching her cheek, letting herself cry, and then moving on.

The Transitioning Problem

Does this sound familiar? You're in a distracting phase, and then you meet a man. There's a mutual attraction, and you begin acknowledging your sexual self. You think about him throughout the day. The anticipation, the hope, makes you slightly more alive, feeling prettier, more open to others. But when you learn the man who sparked your interest is wrong for you, you're trapped. You've awakened your sensual feelings, and now you're exposed without a partner.

Kathleen met Carlos on a three-day bike trip. "Even before he called [after the bike trip], I was cheerier then usual. I loved my normally boring commute; it gave me more time to fantasize about him. I wondered if the man in the next car could see how my breasts were smiling. I felt silly and alive. I must have masturbated more that week than in the prior six months. I paid more attention to how I dressed; I felt more loving, light, and vibrant all week. I love myself when I feel this way.

"We arranged to go biking the following Saturday and had a great time. We went for dinner afterwards. That's when he told me he was married. He wanted to continue seeing me, though, with or without sex! Of course, I said no.

"This whole week I've been an emotional mess. Not about Carlos; I never want to see him again. But I had come sensually alive, and now it hurts to have those feelings again and not have an outlet for them. It's like having gotten emotionally dressed up with no place to go."

Navigating the transition between having your sensuality awakened by a man and letting go of that sensuality without becoming depressed is tricky. In fact, the transitioning is so painful that some women prefer to stay in a relationship long after they know they should end it, and some hesitate to open themselves up with a new one.

The Plan

Consciously using the framework of the three options might have made it easier for Lucille, one of my first clients more than 30 years ago. She was a 32-year-old woman whose husband had walked out on her and her two babies, long before divorce became socially acceptable. Lucille was overwhelmed—taking care of her young sons, working full time, managing her home and her sick father. She had no time, of course, for socializing.

Young and naive, I certainly couldn't appreciate her pain when she said: "It's so awful being horny and not having a man. I wish I could take a pill to make these feelings go away."

At this point in my life, knowing firsthand and from others what it's like having the body raring to go with no available outlet, I dedicate The Plan to Lucille. This tongue-in-cheek plan is to help women make the transition between acknowledgment of and distraction from their sexual feelings, while avoiding the numbness that results from denying them. While The Plan is facetious, impossible to do, the description of it may trigger some useful ideas for handling your own transitions.

The Plan allows women to modulate their sexual feelings by having them close at hand when needed and tucked away when not. Starting on a month with 31 days, you distract your feelings by throwing your passion into other areas of your life. This might be an old hobby or a new venture; you might reach out to different friends; or you might explore aspects of your world you have overlooked. This enriching distraction should deflect your energy from thinking about men and feeling the social and sexual pressure to find a man.

Thereafter, on alternate months, identify the first half of the month as SADs (sexually alert days). On SADs, you are to feel sensual about everything you do. Your daily bodily routine, like brushing your hair, is done with gentle attention to the sensuousness of your motions. On SADs, you actively set out to look for a man—in your old haunts or in new ones. Read the ISOs ("in-search-of" ads); attend singles dances and parties. Ask friends to fix you up. Follow anything and everything that the advice columns and books for singles suggest for looking for a man. Then, during the latter half of the month, unwind and measure the effects, if any, from your efforts before you relax and return to distraction for the next month.

The month of distraction and the half-month of SADs are actually the easy part. As we saw with Kathleen, the most difficult part of The Plan may be transitioning either into or out of the SADs. As you are leaving 31 days of distraction, entering 15 days of acknowledgment, you may have to push yourself to actively seek out ways to meet men. Prepare yourself for hearing those old messages again: "You aren't trying hard enough," or "If you really wanted a man . . ." Be on the alert and protect yourself from a slide into the downward spiral (see Chapter 2).

Then you'll have about 15 days to cope with the transition back to distraction. Over time and with practice, the transition periods will be easier.

My apologies to you, Lucille, that years ago I didn't understand the pressure of your unrequited sexual feelings. The Plan might have helped you, and I hope it provides other single women with an imaginative and improbable way to take control of these feelings. What more doable ways have you found?

Reflection: Tracking Your Sexual Feelings

Using a journal, keep a daily record of your sexual feelings. Pay particular attention to how you move in and out of the different feelings. Do this for a month and see what you are learning about yourself. Here are some questions to help you focus your thinking.

1. Can you tell when you are feeling horny? Can you tell what you do with these feelings? What are the indications when you are acknowledging them? Distracting them? Denying or numbing them? If you feel weepy, self-hatred, or self-blame, note if it occurs more often in one of the options. How do you deal with the transition phase?

2. How do you manage your sexual feelings? Pay attention to when you feel horny. How long does it last? What brings it on? What helps it subside? Can you use the horny energy for other activities in your life, or does it inhibit you, sapping your energy?

Self-Assessment

The fifth task, Hope for Horniness—Facing Your Sexual Feelings, involves four key issues. Look them over to see how you are doing in each one.

Acknowledging Your Feelings

___recognize your feelings
___outlets for sexual release
    ___masturbation
    ___male friend
    ___polygamy
    ___affairs with married men
    ___relationships with women
    ___other

Distracting Your Feelings

___distract your sexual feelings
___recognize the positives of your doing this
___recognize the negatives of your doing this

Denying Or Numbing Your Feelings

___numb your feelings
___recognize the positives of your doing this
___recognize emotional effects of doing this
___recognize the physical effects doing this

Transitioning Between Acknowledgment And Distracting

___recognize how you transition between these feelings
___recognize the positives of how you do this
___recognize the negatives of how you do this

For any category that you are satisfied with, give yourself a "star," either figuratively or literally. For any that you still need to work on, think about what needs to be added or changed in order for it to be satisfactory. Then, write your ideas for that category.

    If you are stuck, talk with friends or family to see how they handle that task. If you are still stuck after that, consider reading a self-help book, taking a course that deals with the topic, or talking with a professional in the area, for example, a sex therapist, holistic medicine practitioner, psychotherapist, or religious counselor.

Men!
Clarifying Your
Thinking About Them

The sixth task for a satisfying single life isn't about men; it's about you. You need to understand the differences between the way men and women communicate in order to distinguish between a man who is inappropriate for you and one who is emotionally available. You also need to know yourself well enough to identify what you need from a man.

Understanding Men

"Why do we women worry so much about hurting a man's ego? When Larry called this evening, why didn't I tell him, 'Sorry, I don't want to go out with you?'"

Joanna is sitting cross-legged on her bed, writing in her journal. The words come spilling out faster than her fingers can move. "Would he really have been crushed? Even if he'd feel awful, why am I more concerned about hurting him than myself, spending time with someone who doesn't interest me?"

Joanna is not a 17-year-old teenager. She is a 37-year-old woman who was widowed in her early 20s. A graduate from a rabbinical school, Joanna had a pulpit for a few years before deciding she prefers to teach.

She stops writing and stares into space, thinking, "I'm a leader in the community, a respected teacher; why am I sounding like a kid?" Then she quickly picks up the pen again to grab her thought. "If enough women were straightforward, maybe men would get the idea there is a problem, do some soul-searching, and seek help. Protecting them may not be so kind after all!"

Are men really so fragile they need to be protected from your honesty? My niece Deborah, who's 28 years old, has found a neutral way to do this. If she doesn't want to see a man again, she explains to him that "dating is like buying a shirt. We need to try each other on for size. If we don't fit, it doesn't mean there's anything wrong with you or me. It's just that we don't fit. We each need a different size."

Deborah's approach is both simple and polite. Joanna could have saved herself many hours of resentment if she had thought about dating in this way. Instead, she continues to question and doubt herself, trying to make a misfit fit.

A few months later, returning from a first date with Manny, Joanna again writes in her journal. "It was going so well, and then he sort of disappeared inside himself. It was like pulling teeth to keep up the conversation. What happened? Was it my comment about the peanut butter? I should have just admired that he was making it himself, not talk about how I used to make it before the days of a Cuisinart.

"On the other hand, maybe the problem started before that. There had been an awkward pause in the conversation, so I asked him to tell me something about himself. Maybe that turned him off."

Do you think Manny is sitting at home wondering why the evening turned sour? Is he saying, "Maybe it was when I . . ." or, "Maybe I should have . . .?" He may not even be thinking about it at all, having just considered it another bad evening. Maybe he didn't think it was a bad evening at all. Joanna worries that Manny didn't enjoy the evening, but more important is that she didn't! Instead of owning her observation, she projects it onto him, making it his thought. (In fact, that wasn't his thought at all, since he called again to ask her out.)

The following week Joanne pursues these questions in her therapy session. "He never asked me anything the whole evening. When he talked about making peanut butter, I may have mentioned how I used to make it, just to give him a chance to ask something of me. Up until then, he had been doing all the talking. Of course, I was asking lots of questions, but if I didn't, we sat in silence."

Joanna catches her breath, and in a voice half an octave lower, she observes: "I'm beating up on myself for how I broke the silence, aren't I? Even here in this room, I'm protecting him and his ego. He wasn't making any effort to keep the conversation going." She takes a few more deep breaths, then slowly exhales. "It wasn't just the silence. He just didn't seem interested in me. In the entire evening, he never once initiated any topic having to do with me."

Joanna is tiptoeing around saying, "I'm not interested in him." Worrying about his ego leads her to accept the blame for an awkward and boring conversation. Why would she (and many other women) do that? As a respected rabbinical teacher and scholar, she wouldn't dream of discounting her perceptions. Why is it different in her personal world?

That night, she again writes in her journal. "Interesting ideas from therapy today. There were many opportunities for Manny to make our conversation into an exchange. I take it all on me, rather than say he's not for me. He has appealing qualities, but he can't carry his share of a conversation; that's important to me. Yet, if I accept that the problems with some of the men I'm meeting are their issues, where does that leave me? They all seem to have some serious problems."

That's what so many women today seem to be saying. Just browse through contemporary cards, newspaper comic strips, magazine cartoons, Internet jokes. By definition, humor exaggerates a point, but these expressions do genuinely reflect women's persistent complaints about men's inability to emotionally relate—whether the men are married or single. If the point didn't ring true, publishers wouldn't print the cartoons, women wouldn't buy the cards. Business doesn't boom for a few disgruntled women.

Women need to stop making excuses for men. As long as, individually, they protect a man's ego, that man doesn't have to face himself. And that makes it easier, collectively, for men to ignore their contributing to and responsibility for correcting problems in relationships.

The Rules Have Changed—For Us At Least

Joanna complains about men. You complain about men. Even your male friends complain about men—they can't talk with them like they can with you. There didn't used to be so many complaints. What's changed?

Women. Women have changed, and in the process they've changed the rules for relationships. Before, the rules were unquestionably clear for both women and men. In fact, the anonymous author of *How to Be a Good Wife,* written in the 1600s, spelled them out, as did the home economic books used in high schools during the 1950s. Simply stated, the rules were: stand behind your man—never beside, and certainly not in front of, him—and put his needs before your own.

As a result of the influences of the women's movement during the past 35 years, women have been rejecting those old rules and writing new ones. Most women today define for themselves what they want and need in a relationship. Most modern-day single women can financially support themselves, and since society no longer calls them "sick, neurotic, and immoral," as a poll in 1957 described them, they can choose to remain single until or unless they meet a man who adds something to their lives. That is, a man who sees and treats them as equals, who listens as well as talks, who tries to understand himself and talks about his feelings.

Kate is an Always Single 38-year-old. As a teenager and young adult, she was always popular with men. She's vivacious, has a winning smile, and exudes self-confidence and openness. She's talking about how things have changed for her over the years.

"I don't mean to brag, but I used to have all the dates I wanted. But now I'm not dating at all, and," she grins mischievously, "it's not because I've gone downhill! I've met some men, but I wouldn't go out with them. Now, within five minutes, I can tell if a man interests me. I'm not too choosy, but I am choosy. When I was in my 20s, if a man presented himself okay and wasn't an ax-murderer, I would go out with him. I didn't know myself well enough to know what I wanted. I didn't know it was important that he show some feelings, that he respect my views. Now, I insist on this, and it narrows my choices."

Men probably aren't that different from 35 years ago; they haven't gotten "worse." It's just that women expect men to adjust to the changes they've made. Many men haven't noticed the changes, however, or they haven't figured out how to adjust to them.

One possible explanation for this has to do with power and patriarchy. While individual men may not feel they have power, men as a group in our society do hold sway in matters of money and decision making—whether in government, business, the arts, or science. As Elizabeth Carter writes in *Love, Honor and Negotiate* (Pocket Books, 1996), we live by the Golden Rule: "The one who makes the gold makes the rules." When you are part of a privileged group, you don't have to make adjustments to please the less privileged. So, it is easier for men to avoid noticing and adjusting to the changes women expect in relationships.

Men Don't Get It

Joanna's statement is powerful: "If enough women were straightforward, maybe men would get the idea there is a problem, do some soul-searching, and seek help." Unfortunately, many single men genuinely don't understand there is a problem.

Shortly after completing the Single Women's study that is the basis for this book, I decided to start a companion study on single men. As a preliminary to that study, I held six group interviews, each group having four to six Always Single and Single Again men, adopting the same format I had used with the women. I was struck that every man talked about wanting "intimacy" and "closeness" with a woman. So, I asked why they were still single.

Unlike with women, there was little self-reflection.

The men didn't look for explanations within themselves. They found fault with the women they had dated, or they assumed they had just not met the right woman yet. Granted, these interviews are not statistically viable, but they do raise some interesting questions.

Large numbers of men aren't being spurred to self-reflection as part of a group movement. And, it appears they aren't doing their soul-searching individually either. Bookstore owners tell me there are fewer self-help books for men than for women, and even those are bought more often by women. This means that women and men have an unbalanced investment in understanding themselves and their relationships.

Men And Women Don't Speak The Same Language

To have a good relationship, women and men both need to be invested in understanding themselves and their relationship. To do this, they need to be at least moderately fluent in the language of the other sex—female-ese and male-ese, as it were. However, even if men don't make the effort to become bilingual, you can. By recognizing gender differences, you are less likely either to blame yourself when something goes wrong or to personalize what men do and don't do.

The information in the box below may help clarify some differences. It has been culled from many studies on gender and shows some of the typical differences in male and female speaking styles. As with all generalizations, they fit many but not all men and women.

In *You Just Don't Understand* (Morrow, 1990), Deborah Tannen describes the differences in gender communication. A man grew up in a "hierarchical social order in which he was either one-up or one-down. Conversations are negotiations in which people try to achieve and maintain the upper hand if they can, and protect themselves from others' attempts to put them down and push them around. Life, then, is a contest, a struggle to preserve independence and avoid failure."

Women, on the other hand, approach the world as "a network of connections. In this world, conversations are negotiations for closeness in which people try to seek and give confirmation and support, and to reach consensus. They try to protect themselves from others' attempts to push them away. Life . . . is . . . a struggle to preserve intimacy and avoid isolation" (pp. 24–25).

Speaking Styles For Men And Women

Men	Women
Speak to report information	Speak to connect with others
Ask questions for information	Ask questions to engage others
Express preference as a definitive	Express preference as a suggestion
In personal discussion, wait for a question in order to know what or how to respond	In personal discussion, assume the other will respond without a specific question
See encounters as a win/lose	See encounters as an exchange of ideas
Must have ideas shaped before speaking	Often clarify ideas while speaking
May abruptly change topic	Connect information to the other's previous comments
Speak louder than the other speaker	Use the same volume (or lower) than the other speaker
More often use "I" and "me"	More often use "us" and "we"
Rarely offer personal comments	Often offer personal comments

Not all conversations between women and men are scrapes between one-uppers and connectors. But in an argument, a man might react to an internal fear of being bested by the woman, while she might fear being rejected by him.

Clues For Understanding Male-Ese

Being bilingual involves understanding the words as well as the nonverbal communication. Here are seven clues that might help you become more fluent in male-ese. (Granted, these are generalizations, but they are useful for women to have as guidelines in thinking about male communication.) They are useful to know, regardless of whether you are in a committed relationship, getting to know a man, or just having to deal with men in your life.

1. Men struggle with shame.

2. Women rapport, men report.

3. Men parallel talk.

4. Men answer questions; they don't ask them.

5. Men like to be helpful.

6. Men yearn for intimacy too.

7. Men avoid fights.

Clue #1: Men Struggle With Shame.

Coming home from a lovely afternoon walk through the park, Carrie says, "Allen, we need to talk." Then, afraid he will walk away or shut her out, she adds—full of affection for him—"Please don't turn away from me."

Allen reflexively assumes she's going to criticize him. He snaps, "You have to ruin everything, don't you. You can't just have a good time and let it be."

Carrie wants to talk about whether they should move in together. Clearly, her loving intention misfires. If she understood the issue of shame for men, she could have started the conversation differently. Rob Becker in his comic one-man show, *Defending the Caveman,* explains what happened. He says those four words, "We need to talk," can send "terror into every man's heart."

Sam Osherson, in *Wrestling with Love: How Men Struggle with Intimacy* (Fawcett, 1992), has a fuller interpretation of Allen's reaction. Chapter 1 is devoted to shame. While shame is one of the most difficult feelings for men to identify and talk about, it also is one that governs much of their behavior.

Osherson lists three ways that intimacy creates shame for men:

1. When they feel they are failing at "manly" tasks, and their self-worth plummets

2. When they get flooded by powerful feelings, usually anger, sorrow, or love, that feel "unmanly" or "ugly" or "defective"

3. When they get in touch with yearnings for connection and contact that seem counter to what a man should feel and how he should behave (p. 32)

Allen also feels the closeness of the afternoon. But for him, these feelings are unmanly. They shamefully stir a yearning that is full of love for Carrie. They put him in the vulnerable one-down position of caring about her so much. He knows that his father would not have acknowledged such deep affection for a woman.

This alone can be confusing for a man. But there is more. When Carrie asks him not to turn away, Allen hears a criticism, which he interprets as an attack. First he feels shame for the strong emotional pull toward Carrie, and then he feels criticized, causing more shame, which makes him want to pull away. He now has several feelings going on simultaneously that emotionally flood him. As a result, he explodes, leaving him feeling worse about himself for having "lost it," a sign of weakness that causes even more shame. This sequence escalates his shame and weakness, characteristics contrary to his self-image.

Osherson continues. "Intimacy creates shame as we confront the painful chasm between our internal idealized images of men as big, competent, autonomous, protective of the weak, and the reality of our human needs and wishes" (p. 32). He goes on to describe typical situations where a man may feel small or incompetent: asking for help, failing at some task, feeling in a one-down position, becoming emotionally flooded, not having the words to express himself. "The bottom-line feeling in shame is that we feel defective, worthless, without value" (p. 32).

Now, let's put together Tannen's ideas about the hierarchical world of one-upmanship with Osherson's ideas about shame and see what happens for Carrie and Allen. Allen hears, "Oops, I did something wrong," and braces for an attack. He assumes whatever Carrie says next will be a complaint, some failure of his. It stirs familiar feelings from when he was little and his father's booming voice demanded, "Allen, get over here." He feels shame for feeling like a child when he's a grown man. Such inadequacy and weakness! And, he thinks, "I don't even know what I did wrong!"

Flooded with all this, Allen explodes. He hears an attack, and he counterattacks. As he later explained: "When someone criticizes or complains about you, you must criticize or complain about them harder. And the one who retaliates the hardest wins." If he can throw the blame back on Carrie, he can hide his shame. So, he finds a way to turn the conversation around so he is angry at her, blaming her for what she did wrong. Now, though, he's ensconced in shame for acting unmanly by getting angry! He's in an emotional maze and nothing he does frees him.

In the same way that many women carry within them the message that their success hinges on finding a man, men carry within them the message that they *should not* be in a one-down position. Which is exactly what so many men feel when talking with a woman about feelings! And that activates shame.

Terrance Real, in his aptly titled men's self-help book *I Don't Want to Talk About It* (Fawcett, 1997), takes this one step further. To ward off shame, men take on a stance of grandiosity. While girls were encouraged to own their feelings and feel connected to others, at the expense of their assertive selves, boys had the opposite internalized message. They were encouraged to develop their public assertive selves, and discouraged from expressing their feelings and making emotional connections with others.

Men are caught in what Real calls "Conditional Grandiosity," which "lies at the core of the male experience. Boys and men are granted privilege and special status, but only on the condition that they turn their backs on vulnerability and connection . . ." (p. 180). This means, Be a winner, not a loser. In order to be a winner, though, they must overpower someone else, but then they are discouraged from feeling for the person they overpower.

They are shamed if they lose, and if they win, they must toughen themselves against physical pain and ignore the feelings of the one they caused to lose. All of this works against experiencing empathy for themselves and others.

But there's more. "Unlike women who are endowed with their being a female, men must have their masculinity bestowed upon them. Our language has many ways of talking about 'becoming a man'" (p. 172). (We never talk about women having to become a female.)

Since maleness is bestowed, it can also be taken away. Men know they must sometimes be a loser. Alternating between the two positions of winner and loser leaves men perpetually anxious about their status as a "man." Grandiosity, then, is the flip side of shame.

In order not to feel like a victim, a man must pump himself to a "falsely empowering position" which, when used with women, is offensive.

The problem for many men lies in the paradox they've been taught: Losers aren't valued among men, so in order to feel accepted, to belong, one must dominate others. Seeing this in the context of relationships, it is amazing that men are able to make any emotional connection with women!

Not all of the men you meet will recognize this struggle, or they might have learned ways around it. It may be useful to you as a woman, however, born with your femininity, to understand what the inner conflict is for the grown-up boys you meet who must continually try to "become a man."

Clue #2: Women Rapport, Men Report.

The purpose of communication is different for men than for women. Using the language from Tannen's *You Just Don't Understand,* communication for women is a form of "rapporting," making connections; for men, it is a form of "reporting," passing along information. Understanding this can explain how a simple discussion can turn into a blowup.

Let's use Carrie and Allen again to see how this works. It's Saturday afternoon, and they are talking about what to do that evening. Carrie asks, "What movie would you like to see tonight?" Allen replies, "How about the new *King Kong* remake?" Instead of offering her own choice—"I'd prefer to see . . ."—Carrie waits. When Allen doesn't specifically ask for her ideas about what movie to see, she reluctantly agrees, "Okay," and then becomes sullen.

At first Allen ignores this, but finally he innocently asks, "What's wrong with you?" She cries (or snaps back) that he doesn't love her; he always gets his way; he doesn't care about her feelings. She doesn't want to see *King Kong*.

Allen is surprised at this outburst. He gently says: "Okay. What movie would you like to see?" But it's too late. Now Carrie feels pacified, like a child. "You're only saying that because I'm upset."

Which is true. Allen really doesn't care which movie they see. From his perspective, Carrie asked him a question and he answered it. He doesn't understand what's happening. From Carrie's perspective, she feels discounted. Her question to Allen isn't meant to solicit an answer to their evening's entertainment. She is opening a discussion. She asks what he wants to see and expects he will ask her in return. That way they each will suggest a movie and then jointly come to a conclusion.

She wants rapport, a sense of connection. Allen, though, is reporting the information that was requested. Not understanding the "rapport-report" communication styles, they each are baffled at how such a simple discussion can deteriorate into an argument.

Clue #3: Men Parallel Talk.

Men "parallel talk"; that is, one man speaks and then the other speaks. They don't give emotive feedback to each other. They don't necessarily pick up on what one says and flesh out the topic. The content of their talk may not even seem related. Let me give you a slightly exaggerated illustration.

Two men are watching a football game on TV.

Man #1: Wow, what a tackle!

Man #2: Did you hear Joe may be going bankrupt?

Man #1: Yeah. That's a shame. Hand me a beer, will ya?

Man #2: Come on, Ref, that was obvious interference!

The men may speak further about Joe in isolated sentences throughout the game. By the time they part company, though, they will feel the comfort of having watched the game together *and* of having been empathic about Joe's financial situation.

Their wives or partners might marvel that at no point did either man say, "I feel so sorry for Joe," nor did they wonder, "Is there something we can do for him and his family?" They may feel the men are being callous and uncaring.

What the women do not understand is what the men unconsciously know: namely, that to do something for Joe would increase his shame by calling attention to his plight. They might also feel shame for openly showing their concern for a friend. When men talk to each other, there's no problem with parallel talk because they speak the same language. The problem occurs when they talk with women.

Clue #4: Men Answer Questions; They Don't Ask Them.

Men don't ask questions. Let me repeat this in another way: men answer questions, but they don't ask them. Everyone jokes about men not asking for directions. Asking is not part of a man's socialization. If you don't know, if you have to ask, you are weak and powerless; you are one-down, and that is shameful.

In general, men don't ask for directions in relationships either. They don't ask, "How do you feel about the argument we had last night?" Or, "I don't understand what you're telling me. Could you try again?" Or, "I don't like it when you start crying and walk away. Isn't there some other way we could handle this?"

If the topic is not threatening, and if it occurs to him, a man might ask questions. For example, Allen might ask, "How much coffee do I put in the grinder?" This isn't an arena where he thinks he should excel.

While men don't ask questions, they nevertheless need women to ask them questions. Men participate better in an emotional discussion if they have something specific to answer. Without that, they may not say anything. While a woman may assume a man is avoiding her, he may say nothing because he doesn't understand what she wants from him. Remember, a conversation is a means of reporting information, so, for him to respond, he needs a specific question to answer.

This runs counter to the female style of communicating. Many women have difficulty being specific; they talk around what they are saying, being diplomatic. They formulate their ideas while talking; or, while expressing one feeling, they get carried along to several others. This can be a problem in a casual conversation as well as in a serious one.

For example, Carrie says, "I had the most unusual day today." Allen may not ask any questions about that because he doesn't think to ask; he may have been distracted and didn't hear what she said; or he may be waiting silently for her to continue. When she doesn't, he might be thinking, "I guess she doesn't want to tell me." However, without his verbally encouraging her to continue, Carrie may feel he doesn't care about her or her unusual day.

In a more serious conversation, Carrie says: "This isn't working, Allen. Maybe we should break up. I don't feel you really care about me. I mean, you spend more time when we're together watching TV or talking about work. You . . ." and she goes on with her litany of complaints. She gives examples. When she finishes, she expects him to have a response. There is silence.

"Well," she asks, "what do you think?"

Totally lost, Allen says, "About what?"

Allen is not playing a game. He really is lost. She has talked a lot, but there is nothing specific he can answer. He needs a question to get him into the conversation.

Clue #5: Men Like To Be Helpful.

"I don't know what to do!" cries Carrie one evening. "My boss is so inconsistent and cruel. First he tells me one thing, then another. It's impossible working for him."

Most women know Carrie wants to hear, "How awful to have to work for such a person." Or, "Your boss should feel lucky he has you working for him!"

Allen cares very much that Carrie is being hurt. In his masculine role of protector, and from his socialization of having to know all the answers, he may feel compelled to solve her problem. "You should tell him . . ." Oops, regardless what comes next, he's committing a critical error!

Carrie, like most women, is smart enough to figure out what to do about her boss or to ask for suggestions if that's what she needs. What she wants here is to know Allen hears and cares about her distress.

By jumping in with suggestions, Allen's effort to be empathetic backfires. Here's when asking a question could be helpful. If Allen asked, "Would you like a suggestion?" Carrie could say, "Yes," or "No," or "Not yet; let me burn off steam first." This way, Carrie would get what she needs—his attentive concern—and Allen would feel appreciated for his caring.

Carrie can avert a bad ending to this situation by not reacting to his suggestions. Instead, she can offer him an alternative response to her. (Chapter 13 goes into more detail on this topic.) For instance, when Allen starts, "You should tell . . ." she might interrupt and say, "I appreciate your wanting to help me with this. So, let me tell you what would help me the most." And then she tells him what she wants to hear.

Another alternative is to wait until some neutral time to have this discussion. However she handles it, if Carrie remembers Allen's intent is to be helpful, not authoritative, she can find less inflammatory ways to react to his suggestions.

Clue #6: Men Yearn For Intimacy Too.

"He's only interested in sex" is a complaint I hear frequently from women. While it may be true for some men, for any man you might consider emotionally appropriate, it's probably not true—even though it may appear to be. In general, a man's style of expressing feelings is governed by his upbringing in a society that assigns gender roles and attributes. In expressing affection, he has been "trained" to do it physically, through his genitals. When he says, "Let's make love," or grabs your breast while walking down the street, or alludes to lovemaking while at dinner, he may be saying, "I care about you." Without understanding this, you may interpret these comments and behaviors as his obsession with sex.

Men need intimacy, and they express that need through sex. They need the sexual contact as foreplay to sharing themselves emotionally with you. Lying in bed in the afterglow of coitus, they are more open to expressing their intimate feelings.

It is exactly the opposite for most women. Women need verbal and emotional foreplay to satisfy their need for intimacy, which in turn stimulates their physical desire for sex. For them, wanting sex is the result of feeling intimate.

One way around this dilemma is to consider the many different ways of making love. Have you ever had an intimate or personal talk with a man only to find yourself sexually aroused—vaginally wet or pulsing? If so, you can see how such a discussion affects you just like physically making love does. Therefore, consider sharing feelings as one way of making love; having intercourse is another.

Thinking in these terms, make a list of other ways you and a man can make love. For example, hiking on a beautiful day, going dancing, playing duets on the piano. Assigning the word *lovemaking* to these other activities may help you both recognize that he is the initiator of making love with sex, you are the initiator of making love in talking, and you both initiate making love in the other ways you've listed.

Reflection: Different Ways Of Making Love

List the different ways you like to make love. Have him make a separate list. Compare them. When you are engaged in the activities on your lists, make sure you use the language of lovemaking.

Clue #7: Men Avoid Fights.

I'm sitting at a long dinner table with middle-aged single men and women, all strangers. A man two seats away is being vulgar toward me through his sexually provocative words and body language. I tell him to stop, several times, in a clear, definitive voice. He persists. Finally, he gets up, very drunk, and walks toward me with puckered lips. He thinks he's going to kiss me! I firmly and politely tell him he's disgusting and leave the table.

Later that night, I ask some of the other men who had been at the table why they didn't step in and tell him to cut it out. It seems to me that that was all it would have taken; the drunk was discounting me, as a woman, but he would have responded to a man's telling him to stop.

The first two men I ask shrug and say I was making too much of it. I should have just ignored him. Another man says I provoked the drunk by even talking to him. All three of these men turned the problem around, making it my fault.

I am dismayed by their responses, but they are easier to discount than Bruce's. When I put the question to him, he thinks for a moment, then confesses, "I didn't want to start a fight."

I catch myself before screaming at him. How can I understand that? I sense Bruce is caring. What in the world can he possibly mean? I was verbally abused and Bruce didn't want to start a fight!

For most men, a verbal confrontation opens up the potential for a physical fight (remnants from the playground). Men don't want to physically fight unless absolutely necessary. Women didn't grow up with the same hierarchical pressure to maintain their position. For them, fighting means arguing, discussing, making someone hear their point. Women tend to press onward where men tend to back off.

Researcher John Gottman has another explanation for this behavior. In *Why Marriages Succeed or Fail* (Simon & Schuster, 1995), he explains that men's physiological arousal rate shoots up fast when they get angered. Therefore, they tend to hold back. Or they explode. There is little middle ground. Women's arousal rate moves up incrementally. This physiological difference accounts for some men's determination not to get engaged in an argument, and for their explosiveness that seems to come from nowhere.

When I saw the situation from inside Bruce's shoes (which was difficult), I could see that for him, and probably all the other silent men at the table, I should have just backed off. They believed I was asking for trouble by confronting the man. By not getting involved, they were avoiding making the problem worse; they believed a physical fight might have ensued if they had stepped in.

On the other hand, every woman at the table, I later learned, was silently rooting for me. They didn't think in terms of a physical fight. They wanted me to let him have it, even if they didn't feel verbally strong enough to confront him themselves.

What Women Need From Men

Joanna is again writing in her journal. "It doesn't seem so difficult, really, to have a healthy relationship. With the right man, I'd be able to use all the skills I've acquired from my reading, thinking, and decades of therapy. We'd share feelings, express our needs directly, speak in 'I' terms, not attack each other. We'd have vigorous but clean arguments. It doesn't seem so difficult, if I only had the right partner!"

Keeping male-ese and the seven clues in mind will make it easier to tell when gender-type language is causing a problem in a relationship, or when it is a case of the man just not being the right partner for you.

A right partner is what I'm calling an emotionally available man, an EAM. There's no one description of an EAM; he's different things to different women. Yet, there are some general characteristics that most women want in a man.

They want him to be:

- bilingual, or at least willing to learn some of the differences between the way men and women communicate;
- emotionally responsive, to hear their feelings and not hide from his own;
- able to tolerate his discomfort with intimacy and not flee from it.

An EAM is not still emotionally involved with an ex-wife or another woman. He is willing to work on a relationship rather than skip out when there are problems. He doesn't blame the woman in order to avoid his share of responsibility for making the relationship work. He's willing to risk and share in the vulnerability of love. He accepts the give-and-take of a mutual relationship, valuing you and treating you as an equal. He appreciates and even encourages your differences.

When you think about whether a man is appropriate for you, you need to look beyond his physical characteristics and his personality to see whether you have similar interests and a chemistry between you. You also need to consider whether he is or has the potential to be emotionally able to have a healthy relationship with you. Both women *and* men feel much better about themselves when they are in a mutually enhancing relationship.

The Ideal EAM Is A Man Who Is:

- bilingual or willing to learn
- able to hear your feelings and express his own
- able to tolerate intimacy
- not emotionally involved with another woman
- aware that it takes *two* to make relationships work
- willing to accept his share of responsibility for relationship problems, not just blame you
- willing to risk the vulnerability of expressing love
- able to participate in the give and take of a mutual relationship
- willing to treat you as an equal
- able to value the similarities and the differences between you two

Your Need List

Those attributes constitute a *general description* of an emotionally available man. You will, of course, have your own specific requirements, such as wanting him to be tall, sensitive, musical, intelligent. Your requirements for a man shouldn't be about him, though; they should be about *you*—what you need from him.

When this topic arose in one of my therapy groups, Linda became quiet and then admitted: "I know what I want *in* a man, but I'm not sure I know what I need *from* him. I don't even know how to go about thinking about that."

Some women are so focused on pleasing a man or on what they want him to be like that they are ill prepared to identify what they need from him. Yet, if you don't know what you need from him, you may not be aware if you aren't getting it.

For example, your "need-from-a-man" list might include:

- listens when I'm upset
- doesn't ignore problems
- doesn't minimize my professional growth
- can tolerate my closeness with my family
- can accept my strong religious beliefs

You might want to further divide your list into two categories: your "top requirements" list would include items that are not negotiable; the other category is "it would be great but not absolutely necessary." Your top requirements might be just one or two items. The other category would include all of the rest of the qualities that are important to you.

By midlife, you are wise enough to know you won't find a man with all the qualities you need, so being aware of your top priorities can clarify what's most important to you.

The main drawback, though, to knowing your own needs is that, regardless of your age, insisting on an EAM may limit the availability of potential partners, making you more aware of the number of men who are *not* appropriate for you. Unfortunately, it may be true that as you get healthier, the pool of appropriate men gets smaller.

On the other hand, the more aware you are of what you need from a man, the less you blame yourself for not being married, and the more choosy you want to be. When you are lucky enough to meet a man who fits your top requirements list—even if he has no other qualities on your list—you will know you have met your kind of EAM.

Why Aren't You Meeting Emotionally Available Men?

Are you responsible for not meeting appropriate men? Don't bother rattling off your personal list of imperfections; men aren't perfect either. Don't bother mentioning your fear of intimacy; everyone has it. Look beyond the quick and easy answers. Are you sending men messages to stay away, *or* is that the explanation you give yourself so you have some control over the problem of not meeting men?

You need to acknowledge the difference between not meeting a man versus not meeting an EAM (or a man with EAM potential). Here are three very different situations.

1. Are you pushing away prospective emotionally available men?

2. Are you not living a life that puts you in contact with men so you don't even have options to see if any of them is an EAM?

3. Are you meeting men but eliminating them as options, based on your being appropriately choosy?

Not Meeting Men Checklist

___ I might meet an EAM, but I push him away.

___ I don't have the opportunity to meet any or many men.

___ I am not interested in the men I meet; they are not appropriate for me.

If you do meet men with the potential for a healthy relationship—that is, if you checked #1—you need to understand why you push away appropriate men. You may need professional help with this.

Don't confuse this with the second possibility—not meeting any or many men. For this, you don't have a problem that requires psychological understanding. You need to find a way to put yourself where men are. If you don't want to do that, that's fine. Be clear that that's your choice, so you don't need to blame yourself for not meeting men.

However, if you do want to get out and be more available to meet men, but you can't, you may need help with *that* problem. The issue isn't that you aren't meeting men; it's why you aren't getting out so you could.

Now, don't confuse these two possibilities with #3. If you are meeting men, but *you* aren't interested in them because they're not appropriate for you, stop beating yourself up for not meeting men. Instead, feel a sense of pride (along with your disappointment) that you are taking good care of yourself by avoiding the wrong men!

Communicating With Men

Even if you are meeting potentially appropriate men, or if you are involved with one, you know that all relationships have communication difficulties. You need to understand how you contribute to them. One of the most common mistakes women make is not being direct: that is, not asking directly for what they want.

Ask For What You Want

Consider these scenarios.

You are all dressed up. You want him to comment on how you look. Ask! Often, men are thinking their compliments but don't think to say them out loud.

You've just returned from giving a presentation. He doesn't ask how it went, not even the topic.

You have an important meeting coming up that you are dreading. He knows you are worried about it, but he doesn't ask how you're doing. You are annoyed or hurt that he doesn't seem to have enough interest in what you are doing. If he isn't asking about you and you want him to, let him know.

Many women believe that if they have to tell a man what to ask, they can't trust his answer. "He's just asking because he was told to do it, not because he really cares." That's not necessarily true. Since asking questions is not a typical mode of communication for most men, they may not think to ask about things that are important to you.

Of course, it is also possible that he doesn't ask because he doesn't care. If he is someone you want in your life, it may be important to you that he begins to care about these things. Therefore, you need to teach him to ask. If he is worthy of you, he'll respond because it's important to you (in the same way you respond to things that are important to him).

There's a difference, though, between asking for what you want and unloading your feelings with words that accuse or blame or hurt: "Talk to me," or its companion, "You never talk to me"; "You take me for granted"; "We don't communicate"; "You never show me you care."

You may feel better for having "unloaded your feelings," but these types of comments only vent your dissatisfaction. They don't state the problem. They are more likely to end a conversation than begin one. They're vague; they don't tell a man what needs to be fixed, and there's no question for him to answer.

Remember, men like to be helpful and to take action, so they need to know the problem or question in concrete terms. Worse, vague or accusatory comments are not only useless, they may also activate a man's shame—telling him he's not doing something right.

John calls me for an emergency appointment. Roxanne, his partner of four years, has just walked out—with her bags. "She says she's told me for two years how unhappy she's been. Believe me, Doc, I never heard her."

How is that possible, you (and Roxanne) may ask? Let's get inside John's shoes. She complains about him, which means he has somehow failed. Feeling shamed, he retreats, which explains how he "never heard her." Each time she complains, he may be reading or watching TV, or he may even be looking directly at her. Yet, he doesn't hear she's upset enough to leave. It doesn't sink in.

Why not? Let's listen to one of their conversations.

Roxanne starts. "I can't stand this any more. You work long hours; you're never here. When you are, your head's still at work. I feel like I'm a piece of furniture for you. [Short silence.] We never go out; you never tell me you love me; you don't comment on how I look. [Short silence.] We rarely make love. I don't know, maybe you have another woman. [Short silence.]"

These silences may be half a second or ten seconds long, but they feel like an eternity to Roxanne as she waits for a response. Getting none, she continues—either out of her discomfort with the silence or from a belief she hasn't been clear enough. At some point, after one of these silences, she cries: "Well, what do you think? Say something!"

Of course, John doesn't.

If, at this moment, we could be inside the shoes of both John and Roxanne, we'd hear something dramatically different. From his perspective, he's just heard a list of complaints telling him he's a lousy man. "She must not love me," he concludes, and remains silent. From Roxanne's perspective, her complaining is not a negative. "I love him enough to want to fix the relationship."

John is the CEO of a major industrial corporation. Certainly in the business world he hears what is said. There the information is presented clearly, with specific goals. There he feels competent. He can fix the problem or choose not to. But Roxanne isn't talking in CEO language.

The relationship problem is not necessarily Roxanne's. But she contributes to the miscommunication with John by not asking directly for what she wants and by not heeding the seven clues for understanding male-ese.

Ask For What You Want—In Bed

When making love, do you tell the man what you like, or do you assume you shouldn't have to? Do you tell him what hurts or is uncomfortable, what is pleasing and erotic, what is distasteful, what turns you on? Most men have bought the myth that they ought to know how to please a woman. It fits in with the masculine mystique that says if there's a problem, the man must figure it out by himself.

Yet, no matter how many women a man has been with, he doesn't know what *you* like. He doesn't know *your* body. The same is true for you; no matter how many men you have been with, you don't know what he likes. The only way he can possibly know what you like is if you tell him! This is a major cause of many relationship problems; an inability to talk about preferences in the bedroom creeps into an inability to talk about other issues, unrelated to sex.

Here's a relatively simple and nonthreatening exercise that may be of help. It entails taking turns in touching all parts of the body in a variety of styles— hard, soft, patting, stroking—and discussing how each stroke on each body part feels. This exercise sets an atmosphere that encourages each of you to ask for what you want. It gets you two talking about preferences, and learning each other's likes and dislikes. There's no right or wrong, no blaming, no guessing, no one-upmanship. It's just identifying your different tastes.

Reflection: Communicating In Bed—Identifying What You Like

Materials: swatches of soft materials like velvet and silk, feathers

1. Choose a place you can lie down, not necessarily the bed.
2. Get undressed down to your underwear.
3. Take turns being the receiver and the doer.
4. Working from head to feet, the doer experiments with different textures on each part of the receiver's body.
   Experiment with soft touches and harder rubs. Use your fingernails as well as the pads of your fingers, both gently and firmly. Go back and forth, in one direction, in circles; go fast and slow.
5. Starting with the scalp, work each part of the face, neck, shoulders, back, etc. Be sure to pay attention to the inside and outside of the upper arms and forearms, the wrists and ankles. Don't forget individual fingers and toes, the tops and undersides of the feet. Avoid genitalia and breasts.
6. The receiver's job is to let the doer know what feels great, good, annoying, or painful.
7. Take your time. This may take 30 minutes to an hour, or even longer. Have fun while doing it; learn more about each other too.
8. You may want to switch positions during the same period or switch on another day. Be sure each has a turn being both doer and receiver.
9. Talk about the exercise during and afterwards.
10. Do not let this exercise end in lovemaking. Keep that separate.

How To Avoid Miscommunication

Here are some tips for avoiding most bilingual miscommunication.

1. Make sure you have his attention before starting any discussion.

2. If you know what you need to hear from him, tell him; don't hope he'll figure it out on his own. This also applies to your having an opinion on a topic. Give it to him even if unsolicited; don't wait for him to ask.

3. In presenting your points, be brief and specific. Condense them to no more than two to three minutes.

4. Use "I" statements. Instead of telling him what he is feeling or doing (no one likes that), tell him what you are feeling about what he says or does. Rather than "You shouldn't ignore me," try "I feel ignored when you don't talk with me in the evenings." Be aware of pseudo-I statements, such as, "I feel you shouldn't ignore me." That's just a "you" statement in disguise.

5. Avoid absolutes like "always" and "never." They tend to inflame and sidetrack you from your point. Stick to the present example and don't bring up old situations.

6. Consider whether you must explain the genesis of the problem, who caused it or why. (Remember, women like to process; men want to problem solve. Likewise, blaming is shaming.)

7. End with a specific question. "Do you see the problem the same way?" "Do you have any suggestions for fixing this problem?" Avoid vague questions like, "What do you think?"

8. Shape your question so it eliminates a blaming battle. Shape it so it offers the opportunity for a solution, such as "What can we (you, I) do about this problem?"

9. Make your point and then stop. Give him a chance to respond. Tolerate the silence as he gathers his thoughts. You may have trained him so that if he keeps silent, you'll keep talking. So, wait.

10. Avoid blame—his and yours. Sidestep his defensiveness or his attempt to draw you into battle.

11. Keep the whole discussion under an hour. If you need more time, set a specific time to continue, later that day or the next. Many men have difficulty concentrating for a long time on an emotional topic, so it's important to keep it brief and focused.

12. Don't let your emotions interfere with what you need to say. Crying, from sadness or anger, may blur your words and distract him. You don't want your tears to become the issue.

13. To be clear about your needs, practice what you want to say.

The box on page 133 summarizes this list. You may want to put it on the refrigerator or bathroom mirror to remind you both of the guidelines for better arguments.

If Roxanne had borne these tips in mind, her conversation with John might have started like this.

"John, is this a good time to talk?" If he says no, Roxanne could ask when it would be a good time, agreeing to talk then. If he says yes, she would continue: "When I suggest ways for us to spend time together, it feels to me that you aren't interested in my suggestions. But more important, you don't offer suggestions of your own. I would like us to spend more time together. Do you have ideas how we can do that?"

She is silent and waits for a response from him. It may feel like an eternity,

Tips For Avoiding Miscommunication

Get his attention

Tell him what you are feeling; don't make him guess

Be brief and specific in your points

Use "I" statements

Avoid absolute terms like always and never; stick to the present situation

End your point with a question (that is shaped to eliminate blame)

Pose a solvable problem, don't just complain

Explaining the cause of a problem may not be necessary

Make your point, then stop

Don't engage in defensiveness; stick to the point

Keep the entire conversation between 30 to 60 minutes

Keep your emotions secondary to your point

Practice in advance

especially if he's come to expect she'll prattle on. When he realizes that's not going to happen, he says in a rising tone: "I can't do anything right for you. You're always criticizing me."

Roxanne should then sidestep his defensive response by responding: "I'm sure you'd also like us to spend more time together. I know we both have busy schedules, but let's put our heads together and find a way to make that happen more often. Do you have some ideas?" She repeats her question, bypassing her chance to rub it in that it is his schedule that keeps them from being together.

The problem has been identified, his defensiveness has been deflected, and John is presented with a specific question to answer.

In the long run, changing the situation is more important than getting the other to confess to being wrong. This follows a business model and is also effective in emotional discussions with men. (See *Dance of Anger* by Harriet Lerner [Harper & Row, 1985] for more specific ideas about dealing with conflict with men. John Gottman's *Why Marriages Succeed or Fail* [Simon & Schuster, 1995] similarly offers insights about arguments that are easily translatable to single women's situations.)

Self-Assessment

The sixth task, Men! Clarifying Your Thinking About Them, involves four key issues. Look them over to see how you are doing in each one.

Understanding The Differences Between The Way Men And Women Communicate

Distinguishing Between A Man Who Is Inappropriate For You And One Who Is Emotionally Available

Identifying Your Need-From-A-Man List

Assessing Your Communication Skills

For any category that you are satisfied with, give yourself a "star," either figuratively or literally. For any that you still need to work on, think about what needs to be added or changed in order for it to be satisfactory. Then, write your ideas for that category.

If you are stuck, talk with friends or family to see how they handle that task. If you are still stuck after that, consider reading a self-help book on communication or relationships, taking a course, or talking with a psychotherapist or pastoral counselor.

10

Grieving

Grieving is a natural and important task for everyone, married or single. No matter how satisfied you are with your life, there are always aspects that haven't turned out as you would have wished. You didn't get into your first choice of a college; you didn't get a particular job; a bid on a house you loved was rejected; you have two children, not the three you wanted; a parent died before your child's birth/graduation/marriage. Life is full of disappointments.

These disappointments, these crushed expectations, don't stop you for long; they don't cause perpetual self-blame. You grieve and move on. In fact, because one door was closed to you, another one opened. Like the speaker in Robert Frost's poem "The Road Not Taken," you take one path and always wonder what life would have been like if you had taken the other—even when the path you did take has been gratifying.

In order to move on in life, you must grieve what wasn't, giving yourself permission to feel the loss. Sometimes the loss is only a momentary "what if"; sometimes it requires deep mourning. Many single women are resigned to the disappointment of not being happily (re)married; some are intensely sad that their life has not turned out as they had dreamed. Regardless of the depth of the loss, you must mourn your lost dreams. This is the seventh task. Only then are you emotionally open to what comes next.

Separating The Wheat From The Chaff

Were you one of the many women raised with the belief that being grown up meant having a loving husband, two or three children, and a white picket fence in front of your home in the suburbs? Valerie did. A petite stockbroker who maneuvers around Wall Street with ease, she was raised by second-generation Japanese parents who adopted and communicated to Valerie the American "white picket fence" dream.

"I was brought up to be a responsible person, and that means being married and having kids, right?"

On Wall Street, there is no question about her feeling grown up, but when confronted with those old internalized messages about men and marriage, Valerie's body seems to become smaller and her voice takes on a childlike quality. "I feel 17, even though I'm far more than twice that age."

My concept of being grown up includes letting go of and coming to grips with what you would have liked your life to be like, and accepting the reality of what it has to offer. In your 20s and 30s, you may still be getting clear about what you do and don't have control over. But by midlife, you've reached what Gail Sheehy in *New Passages* (Random House, 1995) calls your second adulthood. By this point, you probably recognize the differences between what you can change, what you can't, and where you can (or must) make alterations to your dreams.

Margaret, from the study group in Chapter 1, knows that because she has been single for so long, she's had more opportunity to focus on her personal growth without being distracted by dealing with issues of a husband and children. Yet she also knows that "a part of me will only grow within a relationship. So, if I remain single, there's a part of me that will never get developed. But that's okay. If I had married when I was younger, there would be other parts of me that would never have developed. There are advantages to both ways, and besides, you live with what you have."

Many single women dump all of their losses into the same barrel, labeled "I'm single." Doing that, though, leaves you unable to distinguish between real losses and compromised dreams.

Valerie, for example, was terribly upset that she would never have a 50th anniversary party. At 39, with no relationship on the horizon, she probably will not be married to a man for 50 years, and so her sense of loss is genuine.

On the other hand, she was also upset that she couldn't buy a house with a husband—the only way she envisioned having one. This was not a real loss. She simply couldn't separate her wheat from the chaff; that is, she could still have her house, but she'd have to adjust her dream. Her grief over not having her original dream (buying a house with her husband) subsumed her ability to envision any compromise (buying a house without a man).

Single women face at least four types of real loss specific to them. First, there is *ambiguous loss,* the uncertainty about your future because you don't know if you'll ever marry. Second, women can experience *lost dreams,* as Valerie did: a loss carved in the sand of childhood images of what adulthood will be like. Third, when a particular relationship ends, there is a *personal and societal* loss. And fourth, there is the sense of loss that results from *separating your own feelings* about being single from those of the people you love.

Ambiguous Loss

I have adopted the term ambiguous loss from Pauline Boss, author of a chapter by the same title in *Living Beyond Loss,* edited by Froma Walsh and Monica McGoldrick (W. W. Norton, 1991). As a result of her work with families of MIAs (veterans missing in action), Boss gave voice to ambiguous loss—as distinguished from the definitive loss of death—which she later expanded to include a range of non-definitive or unresolved losses.

"A universal task for all families, regardless of cultural diversity, is to resolve loss. For the most part, the larger community helps families do this through rituals at which friends and family gather. But there are also losses that are not given such public validation. The loss is never officially documented or ritualized. A family member may simply be missing, as are hostages, missing children, and MIAs" (p. 164).

Single women might add "missing husbands" because they could be included among Boss's examples. From my study and my clinical practice, it is clear that for many women, the most difficult part of being single is *not* the absence of a man. It is *not knowing* if they will ever marry or have a partner. This ambiguity, along with the absence of physical touch, seems to be the worst part of being single (even for those who love being single).

Single women endure this ambiguous loss, but they always hold out the hope that maybe next week, next month, next year, on their next vacation, at the next business meeting, at the bus stop or the Laundromat, they will meet "him." And the bargaining with the societal messages can proliferate: "I'll try harder"; "I'll start reading the personal ads"; "I'll lose ten more pounds"; "I'll go back to graduate school"; "I'll start therapy."

In the case of a definitive loss, like death, there is no more room for hope or bargaining. You grieve, knowing the person will not return. You reach the stage of accepting that loss. With time, you begin to restructure your world and continue with your life.

With an ambiguous loss, however, there is no definite end point, no validation, no ritual. There is always room for more hope, more bargaining. There is no finality. Therefore, accepting a loss becomes more complex.

Psychotherapists know that helping a woman accept the inevitability of her terminally ill husband's death is usually less complicated than helping a woman whose husband wants a divorce. In the first situation, the husband will die, and she definitely can't be reunited with him. With divorce, there is always the hope that maybe the husband will change his mind; maybe his new relationship will fail, and he'll appreciate what he has in her; maybe if she is nicer, more patient, stronger, thinner . . . The ambiguity is full of maybe's.

Boss says some amount of ambiguity is normal in a person's life, but "long-term ambiguity is a severe stressor and will make vulnerable even the strongest [individual]." When ambiguous loss persists over a period of time, a person "is at risk for becoming highly stressed and subsequently dysfunctional" (p. 167). This only accentuates the credit due single women for *not* being dysfunctional, especially since the larger community offers no support system for women experiencing the ambiguous loss of a husband.

One woman's way around the effect of long-term ambiguity was to stage a coming out party to identify herself as a single woman. Her printed invitations were cute, a take-off on a wedding invitation, inviting friends to join her in celebrating her singlehood. This announcement to the public, the ritual of the party, ended her long-term ambiguity.

If the long-term ambiguity does cause a dysfunction in single women, it most often manifests itself in the form of depression and self-blame. It also may show up in the self-inflicted punishment of obsessive attention to dieting and making the body more appealing to a man (see Chapter 5).

Since there is nothing to do but wait and hope, women suffering from ambiguous loss may become immobilized. They may be stuck in a state of denial, not wanting to believe that they might never find a man. The immobilization may keep them in either the bargaining stage—"I'll lose weight; I'll get more therapy"—or, alternatively, in a state of being depressed.

To be freed from the immobilization of ambiguous loss would entail moving on in their life, to a stage of acceptance. Many women skip the stage of being angry at their situation. Instead, they de-press the anger and turn their feelings against themselves in the form of self-blame or self-destructive behavior: it's their fault they are single.

"I'm really discouraged with this dating business," says 35-year-old Monica. She plops down on the sofa, adjusting her long skirt. "I keep meeting all these awful men. Well, some are okay. I may even really like the man, but it all ends the same." Her voice rises. "They never call back."

This casts Monica, like many women in her situation, into a series of "What's wrong with me?" questions. After grudgingly acknowledging that she's not cold, unemotional, boring, or too pushy, she concludes that even if she were, the men's behavior with her hadn't indicated they'd noticed.

Monica laughs. "But what else could it be? Maybe I just want something I can control; that would make it easier."

"Then you would have something you could work on," I reply. She nods.

Softly I ask: "What if you could look into a crystal ball and see that you'll never meet an appropriate man? What would that be like?"

"It'd be horrible!"

"But," I persist, "if that's what it said, and you believed in crystal balls [she laughs], what would you do?"

"I'd have to stop looking for a man. That would change my whole life."

"How would that change it?"

"I'd have to get on with my life. Now, looking for a man *is* my life." Monica sighs. "I wish I had a man!"

Each of us has probably wished that lots of things in our life were different. You might wish you were taller or shorter, had blue eyes rather than brown, had musical talent. But you haven't spent years trying to change yourself into a 5'9" blue-eyed piano virtuoso! You recognize that that would have been nice, but . . . It is easy to give up these wishes because there is no value judgment, no social or family pressure about changing your height or eye color.

Not having a loving partner, on the other hand, is an ambiguous loss that simultaneously carries with it social and family pressure for you to *do something!* But, by definition, an ambiguous loss means there is nothing you *can do*; you have no control over making it different. Yet, society, family, maybe even you, yourself, believe you should do something about being single.

This presents an untenable bind for some women. They may sound depressed, but that may actually be their de-pressed anger—at being single, at an individual man, or at men in general. Therefore, it is important to consider that it may be the ambiguous loss—the disappointed hope—not the absence of the man that fuels the depression and the de-pressed anger.

I wait until I have Monica's full attention. "If you could meet a man, it would be wonderful. Or, if you knew the crystal ball were correct, you would hate what it said, but at least you would know the future. The hardest part, though, is not knowing which of these two very different paths to pursue. That's what ambiguous loss is about, not knowing for sure whether you'll meet a man, so you should keep on looking, or whether you should just give up and move on."

I certainly have her full attention now. Monica is looking intense, yet simultaneously defeated, as I continue. "I have an idea. How about if we try to make you a bit crazy—following both paths at the same time?"

"What do you mean?"

"Keep on doing what you have been doing—try to find a man . . ."

"Oh! that's so painful. I'm through with those dating matches, personal ads, all of that."

"Well, whatever you want to do about meeting men, continue doing that. But *at the same time,* let's think about how you might live with the ambiguity of not knowing if you will or will not meet a man."

Monica decides to make a list of all the things she has always said she'd like to do some day. She pulls out a notepad and writes the following:

"If the crystal ball is correct, here are some things I can do to fill my time:

- improve my relationship with my sister
- learn Spanish
- finish my master's degree
- go to museum benefits
- buy a condo
- get a cat
- look for a higher paying and more enjoyable job

Monica looks over the list, then adds, "I'd need more friends to do things with; most of my friends now are married."

I watch Monica reading and rereading her list. She looks sad. Finally, I suggest, "Between now and when we next meet, how about putting into action just one of those things?"

To my surprise, she says: "Why do I feel a bit better? I shouldn't. You've just told me to prepare for being a spinster."

"No, I haven't, really. I've just redefined what you are already feeling. You're not clinically depressed; you're struggling with the ambiguity of being single, with an 'ambiguous loss.' I've only told you to be prepared to enjoy what life you now have while continuing to want what may or may not come next. It actually shouldn't make you feel much better." I smile.

"True. I could feel *real* depressed now, couldn't I? It reminds me of my father: maybe I should learn from him. He always wanted my brother to join his law practice. He's never really gotten over his disappointment that my brother went into sales. I guess if he can carry on with his disappointment, I should be able to. But it still hurts. I don't think I'll ever feel good about not having a husband. I want one!"

"Of course you do. And no, you may never get over being sad that you don't have one and not knowing if you ever will. That's life. What you do have to get over, though, is blaming yourself. You've been trying to find something wrong with you to explain why you aren't married. You do have to get over de-pressing your anger. You do have to get on with your other dreams, while waiting."

We can compare coping with death to the concept of ambiguous loss to give some theoretical rationale for what often feels like irrational feelings. Being single in a married world is what Boss calls a severe stressor, making "vulnerable even the strongest." Give yourself credit. Living with ambiguity *is* difficult. When there is no clarity, there is no closure. This makes it harder for Monica, for you, for all women to grieve the loss of the dream and move on.

Reflection: Your Crystal Ball List

1. If you could look into a crystal ball and see that you will not marry or be partnered—ever, or for 15 or 20 years—what are some of the things you would do to fill your time?
2. Make a list of all the ideas that come to you.
3. Group them into categories.
4. Look over the categories. Is there a natural priority of what to focus on first? Or do you just need to take any one item and start to make it happen?

Grief Over Your Lost Dreams

Most little girls start preparing early for their future job of wife and mother. They daydream about their roles and rehearse them with their girlfriends. Do you remember your dreams? Playing house? Pushing your doll carriage? Sharing fantasies about your future husbands and babies while walking to school with friends?

In my elementary school, girls played a game called "Love, Hate, Friendship, Marriage." Based on the letters in our names that matched those of our current boyfriends, we'd learn what type of relationship we'd have with them. We also rehearsed saying our first name with the last names of our boyfriends; I tried Karen Cannon, Karen Bachrach, Karen Reshefsky. We picked our brides-maids (they changed quite often!) and designed our wedding decorations.

What were your particular dreams? Did you have special games to predict your future love life? Can you recall your early fantasies—about husbands, about children? Even if you now are certain you do not want children, these dreams (if you had them) are a part of your past.

Give yourself permission to remember these fantasies. Honor them as part of who you were as a child. Smile as you remember who you were back then and feel good; or cry, or do both, as you reflect on how different your life is now from those early dreams.

One of the things you may *not* remember (or may not have noticed) is how a sentence you have heard numerous times has changed over the years. The inflection in "Do you have a boyfriend, yet?" keeps moving. The six-year-old coming home from first grade is playfully asked, "Do you have a *boyfriend* yet?" Twenty years later, at the weddings of your friends, the emphasis is pushed forward, to "Do *you* have a boyfriend yet?" By the following decade, the stress is on the last syllable, "Do you have a boyfriend *yet?*"

It's important to grieve the dreams of your youth. It's just as important to grieve the loss as you experience it today. Claudia is a short, chubby redhead who wears deliciously colored caftans. She laughs through her tears as she talks about what it means for her not to be married. "I'm warm, loving, sensitive, caring, intelligent, active. (I sound like a personal ad, don't I?) I really *am* all these things! Plus, I love being in a good relationship; *I love loving.*" She smiles as she says this, then gazes out the window for a long minute. She watches a male robin bring food back to an expectant mother in a newly built nest in the oak tree adjoining the building. Claudia sighs, "I can't believe I may never be with a man again!"

Yvonne's grief, by contrast, spans her history. She recounts an incident that occurred the previous week.

"I was just lying there, listening to the radio. I was feeling so good. You know how your mind can jump from one thought to another, with weird associations? I was listening to the radio and thought about Howard's radio. Mind you, we've been divorced for almost 19 years. The first thing each morning, he turned on the bedroom *and* bathroom radios. I liked knowing someone so well that I knew his routine. I don't have anyone like that in my life now, and I probably never will again.

"Then, a few minutes later, it really hit me. Howard was 19 years ago! Has time really moved that fast? I finally got out of bed, but I was so sad—not that we divorced, but that time has moved so fast . . . and I am still alone."

Existentially, everyone is alone, but for some women, in some core place deep inside, your aloneness without a man is scary. You don't talk about it for fear of sounding "desperate," or because you know it would just sound like you're lonely for a man. *You* know, though, that there's a huge difference, that it's something more than can be described with words. It's a powerful visceral feeling that sometimes causes you intense grief or terror. Most of the time, however, it stays safely tucked away under the thick covers of your self-confidence and self-assurance that you can live a full life without a man.

Women in my study voiced a range of feelings about being unpartnered. Before you read some of them, though, understand that these are the comments of competent and capable women who are leading active lives. They aren't women who go around moaning about not having a man. In fact, for some, their close friends do not even know how intensely they hurt. If you don't keep this in mind, you might read these sentences as if they were from lonely, depressed, desperate women. They definitely are not!

I'm wasting my womanhood. I have so much to give.

I feel cheated. Not from not having a husband as much as that I won't be able to experience the wonderful feeling of loving and being loved.

I've gone as far as I can go alone. Now I need to be with a caring man, to see if I can have an orgasm *with* intercourse.

Why aren't I married? I'm just as good as the next woman. I deserve to have a man. What's wrong with me? No, I must catch myself; there is nothing wrong with me. But, it's not fair. Other women have a husband, women who aren't as smart as me. Women who haven't spent the years I have in therapy, learning more about myself. Why aren't I married? It just doesn't make sense!

I can't stand it! I can't believe I'm 45 years old and crying about the same things as when I was 30. Fifteen goddamn years. Then I go blank and don't feel anything.

I get so sad after a really wonderful fantasy. I imagine a loving man who can really "talk" with me! He becomes so real. I have designed such a healthy relationship that I get more depressed afterwards because he's not here with me. I carry him around inside me as if he were a real person, expecting him to come home in the evening. When he doesn't, I get more depressed, as if I have lost him.

I'm a kisser. My lips are going to waste.

Reflection: Grieving Lost Dreams

1. Write down this question: "How do I feel not having a loving committed partner?" Now try to answer it, being as honest as possible. Give yourself permission to dip beneath the surface, under your public facade. This may be a difficult task. You may worry that if you acknowledge your feelings, you'll have to feel the sadness you've tucked away in some private place. (As one woman said: "I've put my feelings in a box. Why pull them out again?")

2. Review what you wrote; are there any surprises? Did you say more than you had known you felt? Did you add new ideas?

3. Now, write this question: "What do I do with these feelings?" Again, in answering, be as honest with yourself as possible. You may need a few days or even weeks to accumulate this list. (For example, "I eat." "I work late nights and weekends so I don't have to feel them." "I obsess about finding a man; that's better than feeling desperate about growing old alone." "I work out at the gym." "I throw myself into my painting." "Menopause takes care of most of my feelings.")

4. Assess your list. Are you content with your answers? With how you handle your feelings of not having a partner? If yes, pat yourself on the back. If you've listed items that you don't like, think about what you can do differently.

5. Periodically, you may want to revisit this exercise and compare your responses.

The Grief Circle

Every week, Jennifer takes the largest chair in my office but draws herself into the far-left side. The chair looks lopsided, like it might tilt over. She speaks in a tiny voice and barely moves her body. When asked about this, she is aware it's in sharp contrast to how she presents herself at work, with friends, in the rest of her life. I wonder: "What is it that causes her to shrink here in therapy?"

Jennifer initially sought therapy because she has what she describes as a low-grade depression. It doesn't interfere with her life, and her friends don't even know, she says. But it is getting harder to keep it under wraps. "Besides, I'm tired of always feeling this way."

After a few weeks, when nothing she has said can account for her depression, the absence of the topic of romance—with a man or a woman—stands out in bold relief. When I raise it, within seconds she is sobbing. "I try not to think about it because when I do, I can't stop crying."

We talk about her life and her feelings about being single. She is comfortable in her home, has good friends, a rich spiritual life, and several outside interests. In fact, "If it weren't for not having a man, I'd have a very good life," she wails. "But I'd give it all up just to have a man."

Incredulous, I challenge, "You don't really mean that, do you?"

"I know it sounds awful, and I would hate for anyone else to hear me say this, but I can't stand how I feel. I can't stand the thought of never having a man. If that's what it'd take, I'd do it quick as this." She snaps her fingers. The power and authority of her voice stand in stark contrast to how she usually presents herself.

We need to try something different. I give her a sheet of colored paper and a basket of magic markers and crayons. I ask her to draw a circle showing the size of her pain. Pressing hard with the black marker, she draws a thick circle consuming every inch of the paper. I ask her to show me, using another marker, how much of that pain belongs to others. She looks blankly at me. When I repeat the question, she says, "I don't understand; it's all my pain."

A woman sometimes unconsciously carries feelings, especially anger and sadness, for those she loves—carries them as *if they were her own*. This means that she feels her feelings together with someone else's. As a result, her intense grief (or rage) is enormous because she is carrying a double load.

Sounds weird? Not really, when you consider that women typically are conscientious about not wanting to see someone they love hurting. It's as if in the middle of the night her unconscious gets together with her loved one's unconscious over a cup of tea and says, "Let me carry your sadness (or anger) because I know it's too painful or heavy for you."

I gently push Jennifer. "Think more carefully; some of this huge circle of pain is yours, but can you show me how much of the pain belongs to your mother, how much to your father, how much to others?"

"It's all mine," she insists, sounding slightly defensive.

"Would you mind just holding the marker and thinking about whether the circle can be divided in some way?"

Jennifer carefully replaces the black marker and picks up a thin green crayon. After a few minutes of silence, she draws the following picture:

When she is finished, she stares at the paper, looking surprised. "Not only can I divide the circle, but look at what a small portion belongs to me!" There are

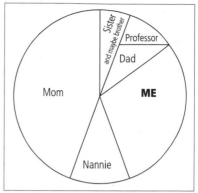

Jennifer's Circle

six slices to her circle. By far, the largest section—about 50 percent—is marked Mom. There are two slices of about equal size. One is for Nannie, her mother's mother; the other is divided into three sections: her sister, an English professor, and her father. The balance, about 25 percent of the whole circle, belongs to Jennifer. In this section, she has drawn the word *me* in thick, dark letters.

"I can't believe this. I never even thought about it. You mean, I may not be as sad as I think I am? That's odd."

We begin talking about giving back to others their sadness about her being single, letting them take responsibility for their own feelings. She practices conversations she might have with each person in the circle, how she would broach the subject, and what she would say to each. "I don't really need to talk to my English professor. Just seeing it here makes it clear how silly to feel obligated to her for something she said to me many years ago.

"It won't be difficult to talk with my sister, but I do need to think about how to raise this with my father, Nannie, and especially my mother."

I remind Jennifer: "The conversations need to be about *their* feelings about your being single. You don't need to defend yourself. You also don't need to convince them of anything. You just need to give them each a chance to say, out loud, to you, what they are feeling about your not being married."

Less than two months later, Jennifer has made a special trip to visit her parents and another to see her grandmother. She's amazed. The conversations went better than she had expected. Nannie didn't really understand anything she said, but "*I* felt better just for having talked to her. I'm not sure how much my mother understood what I was saying, but again, *I* felt better for having talked with her, hearing what my being single means to her. I actually had a great talk with my father and learned about his aunt who never married."

Jennifer is sitting square in the middle of the chair now. "You know, I still am sad. No, I'm angry now. Angry that I'm single. I can't stand the thought I may never marry, but something feels different now. I feel a bit freer; I don't feel like I'm walking around with a ten-ton weight inside. I don't start weeping at the thought of not having children or when I see a couple holding hands. I feel sad, almost wistful, but not that awful feeling I used to have."

Jennifer has finally come to grips with this stage of grieving a loss: namely, anger. As she stops de-pressing her anger, she can stop other self-destructive feelings like self-blame and perpetual grief. Having returned the parts of the sadness that weren't hers, she feels freer, lighter. While she still has her hope, she is in touch with her anger at not being married. (See Chapter 15 for constructive ways of using your anger.) Her grief, though, is a more manageable weight and doesn't interfere with her daily life.

Reflection: Grief Circle

How can you tell if you are carrying someone else's feeling? You might want to try this exercise.

1. On a large piece of paper, draw a circle representing the size of your sadness or grief about being single. You might fill the whole page or only part of it. Be honest. No one else has to see your drawing. Look at the circle to make sure it really does represent the full size of your pain.

2. Divide the circle into as many sections as there are people affected by your being single. You may need space for siblings, grandparents, aunts, uncles, godparents, cousins, neighbors, teachers, religious leaders, society. Don't forget people who may be deceased. Your list is uniquely yours.

3. Use a separate sheet of paper for each person on your list. Jot down ideas of what you need to say to each person who's a part of your circle. Later, you may want to talk to them in person or write them a letter. (For those who are dead, have a silent conversation with them in your head.) Remember, the point of your conversation is to get them to talk about their feelings about your being single.

Crystal Ball

I have heard many women say, "If only I knew for sure, I'd know how to get on with my life." In an effort to help women deal with ambiguity better, to sidestep those messages, I ask women, "If you could look into a crystal ball and see for sure that you will never have a committed long-term relationship, or you won't meet this man for another 15 years, what, if anything, would you do differently with your life?"

In one group where I asked this question, Chris answers first. A large-boned tall woman, she looks like she'd prefer to be outside on a playing field or hiking trail or anyplace other than my office at this moment. "It would be terrifying. It would change my life . . . not to hope any more." She shifts in her seat and plays with a button on her shirt. "Yet, I think it'd be a relief, too. I'd love to give up thinking about it."

Eve's looks are as different from Chris's as is her answer. She's tiny and has flowing blond hair pulled back with a Flintstone barrette. "That's why we don't have crystal balls. Who'd want to give up hope? That would be awful!"

"That wasn't the question," retorts Chris. "It was if we *did* look into one, and if we *knew* what was ahead. The more I think about it, the more I'm sure I'd be thrilled. I could relax. I could think about what I'd want to do with my life. I could concentrate on other things, taking the time I put into finding men for my own interests."

Charlene is looking around the room as if trying to read the reactions on the faces of the other women. She's tense; her words come rushing out. "I'd be real scared. I'd have to change my whole way of looking at things. It'd be hard and sad. But, it'd take the pressure off." She stops to catch her breath. When she speaks again, it is slowly, without the strain in her voice. "I'd do things differently. I'd develop other friendships, travel. I'd be real sad, but then I'd get busy with my new life."

When ambiguous loss gets in the way of your developing all aspects of your life, you might find the "icing" concept from *Flying Solo* (Anderson & Stewart, 1995) to be helpful. View your life to be like a rich chocolate cake. If you meet a man who is right for you, he's just the icing on an already delicious dessert.

The crystal ball exercise is an opportunity to figure out what is really important in your life, what gives your life meaning. Then you can set about making it happen. If a man appears, he will fit into your ongoing full life; if he doesn't, you are left with a full life of your choosing.

Personal And Societal Grief

In addition to your lost dreams of how life should have been, you may be experiencing a personal loss of a particular man. When a relationship ends—whether a man you love or a man you are just getting to know—you may feel genuine grief. The pain is for the three-part hole left by his absence. You may grieve the loss of his company, the loss of the physical and sexual contact, and the loss of whatever degree of emotional closeness existed or was developing.

You may also experience a social grief, mourning the absence of more men who are capable of emotional closeness. Unlike divorce, there is no recognized ritual for mourning these types of losses. You may continue to live with a low-key sadness. Remember, though: recognize and validate your grief, but *do not* blame yourself. *It is not your fault!*

Parents' Grief

Your not having a husband or children defines your life, but it also defines the lives of others. Parents, siblings, close family friends—each of them correspondingly loses a role, either as grandparents, aunts, uncles, in-laws, godparents. Those who experience the loss of such a role may turn to nagging you to try harder to find a man, or they may criticize you for being too fussy. They may try to introduce you to someone you'd rather not meet. While they love you and want you to be loved, this pressure and criticism has more to do with them than with you.

It's Sunday morning, about 11:00. One of the small groups has been meeting for about an hour. The topic at this point is, "Do you feel pressure from your parents, directly or indirectly, to be married?" The stories the women are sharing get punctuated with much laughter. April is sitting with her back to the window. The sunlight slices across her ebony face, accentuating her dancing black eyes. When it is her turn, she shifts in her chair so she can talk using her whole body. She's recounting a situation that happened a couple of years ago.

"I got a call from Aunt Ethel asking me to meet her for lunch. I was delighted because she was always my favorite aunt, but I hadn't seen her for some time. We met at a little cafe we used to visit when I was a child. It's run down now, but the food is great, there's lots of privacy for talking, and it harbors all these special memories for me.

"After we order, Aunt Ethel says, 'You remember Little Perky? You used to go to primary school with him.' I cautiously nod my head, curious where this conversation is leading. 'His wife died from cancer,' she says, somehow looking both solemn and excited at the same time.

"'Should we send flowers?' I ask, knowing I'm making this tougher on her.

"'Well,' Aunt Ethel's excitement is quickly fading, 'you knew his wife.'

"It's now clear where this is heading. I interrupt her, partly to save her from more discomfort and partly from my growing annoyance. 'What do you want me to do? Go to the coffin and . . . [April leans down, pantomiming as if she is touching the dead body.] Oops, she's dead.' [Pantomiming turning to Perky.] 'Perky, we went to school together. I'm sorry she is dead, but I'm alive. Want to get married?'"

The room shakes with laughter, and we never do learn how Aunt Ethel reacted. Although April is a funny storyteller, the pain of the story is not lost through the humor. April was greatly pained at her aunt's well-meaning but nonetheless intrusive suggestion.

Why do families meddle? Is it just nagging or is there something else? If you focus only on how much you hate what they're saying, you may overlook something important *about them*. For example, Aunt Ethel has no daughters of her own; she desperately wants to be a grandaunt to her favorite niece's child.

Your singleness may be causing your parents real grief, for you *and* for them. They may feel guilty for what they think they did wrong, or they might worry about who will take care of you after they're gone. Unfortunately, instead of talking about how they feel, they may offer you suggestions on meeting men instead.

One way to defuse these types of unpleasant encounters is to speak the unspeakable. Can you imagine asking your mother and your father, separately, how they feel about your not being married? Consider, for a moment, how you would feel doing that. What responses could you anticipate? Are they more concerned about your not having a loving partner or your not having children?

Fathers often worry that their daughter will not have anyone to take care of her. You know you don't need to be taken care of, but your father may be a product of his socialization, which says he is supposed to take care of you until he hands you over to a husband. Your father may also feel the loss of the continuation of his family line. If you don't marry and have children, his heritage ends.

In addition, he may be looking forward to the opportunity to be a better grandfather than father. Now he may feel wiser, more patient, and less stressed about work. He may have had a positive role model in his own grandfather and grieves his inability to play out that role for his grandchild.

Similarly, a mother may feel terribly sad that her daughter is not being loved by a man, knowing (because she had it or didn't have it) how wonderful it is to be loved like that. In addition, as females, mothers may absorb the responsibility for having caused you to be "unmarriageable." This is fed by a cultural tendency to blame a problem on something the mother did or did not do. Mothers may also feel your not marrying is a way to punish them for not being a good enough mother.

If you can help your parents talk about what they're grieving—for example, their loss or their self-blame—they might stop hounding you with suggestions for meeting men or criticizing you for not meeting them.

If your parents are concerned about your not having a child, try to understand what that means to them. Ask them! For your mother, it may be her sadness that you won't experience the joy of having your own child. She may be recalling her pregnancy or the early years of her parenting. It could also be her grief about the loss of her own next role. Your not having a child may mean she won't be a grandmother.

In some cultures, being a grandparent is a sign of status: the more grandchildren, the higher your status. In addition to status, conversations among many seniors often revolve around children and grandchildren. You may be depriving your mother and father of a major source of communication; they may feel left out when their friends get together. They may feel their friends pity them (or you) for not being married and having children.

Both your parents may be looking forward to making amends, being better grandparents than they were parents to you. Also, not being a grandparent may force them to think in terms of their own finality—if they can't think about your bringing in a new generation, they may have to think about their own generation's mortality. Listed below are some topics for conversations to have with your parents, individually and together.

Father	not meet his responsibility to give you away in marriage to a man
	not have a grandson to pass on his name and heritage
Mother	blames herself for your being single
	feels sad you are not being loved
Parents	not able to move to their next life stage
	worry about your being alone in your old age
	embarrassed when they can't join in as their friends talk about their grandchildren
	have to focus on their old age if they can't be distracted by a younger generation (your children)

For these and many more reasons, it's important that you talk to your parents. Does the thought of such a discussion cause you indigestion? If so, why? Do you fear opening a Pandora's box—if you give them an opening, they'll tell you all you're doing wrong? Not if you handle it well and keep it focused on *their* reactions to your being single. Besides, you are already dealing with their reactions anyway, only not overtly. Getting the conversation out in the open will make it easier for you in the long run. You will know what each of them *really* means when they complain about your not being married, not combing your hair, wearing shabby clothes, not making enough money, etc.

Most misunderstandings in families are because people merely say part of what they mean; they do not want to hurt the other, so they swallow their full intent. Yet, that frequently is the very thing that makes matters worse.

Your mom and dad probably have visions of how the world should be—based on their dreams for you and themselves. When they react badly to your lifestyle or behavior, it may be because it affronts something personal for them. If you try not to take your parents' reactions personally, if you try to hear them talking about *their own loss,* it will help you depersonalize their reactions. It also may defuse a potentially unpleasant scene.

Let's assume you believe your not having children is what causes your mother the greatest pain. Consider this scenario:

Daughter: Mom, I know you have really looked forward to being a grandparent to my child. You have told me about the dresses you want to buy my little girl and the clothes you want to make for her dolls. You're so wonderful, you even look forward to babysitting her! I know my having a child is important for you, so I know my not being married makes you very sad.

Mother: Well, you'll get married soon. You just need to try harder to stop being so fussy. You always find things wrong with men. You need to . . .

Daughter: I'm sorry for interrupting, but it doesn't feel good when you tell me what's wrong with me. The fact is that I am not married because I haven't found anyone I want to marry. I feel sad about that, and I know you do too. Tell me, Mom, what is the worst part for *you* about my not being married and not having a child?

Note how the daughter cuts off the unwanted comments while still being empathic to her mother. She also acknowledges that she feels sad. This puts the issues out front, and then she immediately switches back to having her mother speak about her feelings. It is respectful while also being self-protective. It gives her mother a chance to talk about what she probably has not verbalized fully to anyone—even to herself.

Listen carefully to see if you can figure out what your mother's main feelings are. Is she guilty, as if it is her fault? Does she feel helpless because she can't find you a husband? Remember, some mothers put pressure on themselves to be able to solve all of their children's problems. Have a similar conversation with your father, who probably has different feelings. Don't assume one conversation will do for them both.

Not all single women are grieving, but for those who are, it helps to separate the different issues. What do you feel about not having a husband? About the ambiguity of never knowing if you will? What do your family members feel? By keeping these issues separate, it becomes easier to see whose feelings are whose, and which ones are giving you more trouble than others. Putting this in perspective can help turn what may have seemed an overwhelming and unending grief into something more manageable.

If Valerie had done this, she'd be sitting in her new home now. She'd be musing over the reality that she'll never have a 50th anniversary party while planning a housewarming party!

Self-Assessment

The seventh task, Grieving, involves five key issues. Look them over to see how you are doing in each one.

Making Distinctions Between Real Loss About Being Single And Compromised Dreams

Recognizing Your Ambiguous Loss

Identifying Your Lost Dreams

Separating Your Loss From Others' Feelings Of Loss

Preparing For The Message Of Your Imagined Crystal Ball

For any category that you are satisfied with, give yourself a "star," either figuratively or literally. For any that you still need to work on, think about what needs to be added or changed in order for it to be satisfactory. Then, write your ideas for that category.

If you are stuck, talk with friends or family to see how they handle that task. If you are still stuck after that, consider reading a self-help book, taking a course that deals with the topic, or talking with a professional in the area, for example, a psychotherapist or religious counselor.

11

Making Peace With Your Parents

Thomas Wolfe said you can't go home again, but he was wrong. As an adult you *must* go home again, literally or figuratively, so you can meet your parents as an *adult*. You must go home again so you can free yourself from falling back into the child role when you are with them, or even just thinking about them. You must go home again, regardless of whether they are deceased, or they are so cruel you don't ever again want to be in their presence. You must go home again so you can be the adult you want to be—with them and with others.

You Must Go Home Again

The eighth task for a satisfying adult life is coming to grips and finding peace with your parents. This means understanding what led them to behave the way they did, letting go of any debilitating anger and resentment you feel toward them, and finding ways to maintain *some positive connection* with them (even if only in your mind), which does not necessarily mean offering your forgiveness.

Growing up and leaving home, psychologically, is a lifelong process, totally unrelated to removing your physical presence from your parents' home. It has nothing to do with how old you are or even if your parents are still alive.

In order to do this, you must first understand the rules and the invisible loyalty that continue to bind you to them. Then, you need to be able to go back home—that is, to resolve unfinished business, whether in your head or in reality—so you will be psychologically free to leave and literally visit as you wish.

Unpacking The Suitcase

Everyone grows up with emotional baggage—unresolved issues from childhood, old hurts and resentments toward your parents. We've absorbed from our parents an unspoken set of rules for living and relating to others, some of which are positive and some of which are destructive. Since they are unspoken, we may not even know we are still bound by them. You may think you've left them behind, but they have an insidious way of reasserting themselves in our daily lives. Therefore, by adulthood, we may be dragging around an exceedingly heavy suitcase.

But, you protest, you've put all that stuff behind you. You are living your own life now. Maybe. But ask yourself: Have you ever said you'd never be like your parents, only to see yourself repeating those very traits you dislike? Do you find yourself arguing with your siblings over the same topics or in the same style your parents used with each other? Do you have friends or lovers whose behavior reminds you of your parents' worst qualities? Or who bring out those qualities in you? If you answer yes to any of these questions, it suggests that the old patterns have continued into your adulthood, and the old family rules are still intact, leading you to find your mother, father, and siblings in your adult relationships. (For more on siblings, see Chapter 12.)

You can't undo the bad experiences from your childhood, but you don't have to drag around the effects like unwanted baggage. My good friend and colleague Susan Wooley has played with the suitcase image. She suggests you should carefully sort through your suitcase to see what's in there, then decide what you no longer need or want to carry with you. Don't be surprised if you feel a sadness at leaving behind some of the old belongings—family rules and behaviors—even though they no longer fit who you are, even if they are dysfunctional. You wore them for years, so you may have a lingering affection for them.

Family Rules

All families have rules. They are deeply programmed, unwritten, and rarely verbalized. They act as trances for the whole family. There are rules about what roles you must play within the family, such as the troublemaker, the comic, the successful one, the peacemaker, the good little girl. There are rules for social behaviors; in many families the "responsible" adult gets married and has children.

There are rules about what you can see and when you must be "blind," like not noticing mother's mental illness or father's alcoholism. Rules dictate what topics—such as incest or illegitimacy—must remain cloaked in silence and secrecy. There are rules about anger and how it's to be expressed. In some families, it is acceptable to yell, while in others, anger can only be expressed indirectly through passive aggression or withdrawal. There may be rules about closeness, and whether it is or isn't acceptable to openly show affection.

Certain rules—when you are in trouble, you can turn to your family; it's okay to like your siblings— enhance family loyalty. On the other hand, dysfunctional rules—don't trust men; women are weak—can erode a family's well-being. From early childhood on, you are learning and absorbing the rules of your family.

Reflection: Identifying Your Family Rules

1. Make a list of the rules you directly heard while growing up, as well as the ones that were implied. These are rules about how you should behave, what you should value. This is probably not a list that can be done in one sitting. More ideas may arise throughout the week—as you catch yourself acting according to them.
2. Check with your siblings. See if they can remember some you haven't considered.
3. Group the rules under different categories, such as anger, sex, money.
4. Using different color magic markers, highlight the positive rules you want to perpetuate and the negative ones you want to remove.

Growing up means unpacking and sorting through your suitcase of family rules, honoring and keeping the ones you like and jettisoning the destructive ones. It means breaking free from your family's trance and seeing yourself and other relatives more realistically. It means making your own rules for living according to your own values.

Defying your parents and choosing a different lifestyle from theirs is rebelling against them; it's reacting *to* them, rather than freely choosing a life for yourself. In the same way, you are not free (or grown up) if you acquiesce and accept their expectations and rules. These are two sides of the same coin: rebel or acquiesce. Both are *in reaction to* parents. They don't leave you free to make your own rules, separate from parental influences.

When you are truly free, you may end up with some of the same rules as your parents, but *not because* you've blindly accepted theirs. You may reject some of their rules, but *not because* they are theirs. You make your own rules because they are right for you.

When Beth first walks into my office, I'm struck by the mixture of expressions upon her face: sadness and bitterness vie for space with a contagious grin. Her eyes quietly laugh. As she tells her story, though, sadness dominates.

She and Carter had been long-time friends before they married. They waited ten years before they had their two children. When their oldest daughter was 15—the age Beth had been when she and Carter first met—Carter confessed to an affair and Beth told him to leave.

Beth threw herself into mothering and her job as a telecommunications analyst. Five years later, even though divorced, she is still depressed about Carter's betrayal. In a moment of insight, the grin briefly asserts itself as she reflects, "It's like I *need* my depression." Then the grin disappears.

When I ask why, the sadness pushes to the forefront. "I never wanted to be like her [Beth's mother]. She was so depressed my whole life and so mean to me. [Family rule number one: We're not worthy of being happy or loved.] I can't believe this is happening to me."

Beth goes on to describe how she grew up hearing her mother constantly complain about her father. "True, he was weak, depressed, and not worthy of her. But she was bitter my entire childhood. She could have divorced him, but she never did. She never got therapy; she just complained. Even since he died—and it's been 20 years now—she has continued to feel resentful. [Family rule number two: You must remain stuck and unhappy in life.]

"She's a miserable old lady." Beth sighs heavily. "Yet, look at me. I'm a mirror image of her!" One tear silently rolls down her left check. In addition to being shackled to her family rules, Beth is caught in an invisible loyalty to her mother.

Bound By An Invisible Loyalty

Family loyalty can be a strength that enriches family members with a sense of connection and support. Or it can be a shackle that binds you throughout life. Loyalty carries an "obligation to belong" and a demand to stay connected that reach out prior to birth and beyond death. Children who have never known their birth parents feel a loyalty to them as well as to their adoptive parents. This is true even if they have never shown an interest in the people who gave them life. Even the deaths of your parents may not free you from the invisible ties that bind you to their expectations for you and their belief systems.

Loyalty goes beyond the quality of their parenting. Whether your parents were loving or cruel, cared about you or neglected you, your obligation to belong to them is tight. You stay connected throughout your life to the parents of your childhood either through positive *or* negative loyalty.

Part of growing up involves confronting *your choice* of loyalty and the family's stated and unstated rules. It includes stretching beyond the world as they defined it for you in childhood and expressing your own ideas.

If you are lucky enough to have had a reasonably good relationship with your parents while growing up, to have felt loved, then you know that their mistakes in raising you were a result of their limitations, not their ill will toward you. Because of invisible family loyalty, the normal separation that accompanies growing up—questioning parents' rules and beliefs—may leave you feeling like you're abandoning them. It may feel disloyal to knowingly hurt them, knowing they will feel rejected if you establish yourself as an adult who differs from them.

Even if you don't like your parents, the obligation to belong is strong and demands loyalty. If you are one of the less fortunate women who come from a dysfunctional family, you must still contend with loyalty—your negative loyalty. Your parents may have been subtly or blatantly cruel; their behaviors may have intentionally harmed you. They may have been physically, sexually, emotionally, or verbally abusive to you or to some other family member. They may have emotionally abandoned or neglected you (such as through their alcoholism or mental illness), or literally have abandoned you. You may have grown up ashamed of your family, shrouded in a secrecy that separated you from your friends.

The more destructive the home, the more intense the desire as you grow up to cut yourself off from your parents. Fleeing (literally or emotionally) often seems the only solution to remove yourself from their negative influence. You might think cutting yourself off from cruel parents would be an act of freedom, a necessity for your emotional survival. But adult children of even the most abusive or unloving parents also struggle, usually unconsciously, with feeling disloyal as they separate themselves from their parents, choosing a life without cruelty or with affection. To be successful at that is to really abandon your parents.

Beth, not having gotten the nurturing she needed as a child, cut herself off from her mother, first emotionally, and for the last eight years, physically—no visits, no calls, no letters. She thought that if she didn't talk to her, didn't see her, she wouldn't have to deal with her.

Here she is, living across the country, trying to remove all vestiges of her mother from her life. Yet, she still must face the reality that she's re-created her mother's life through her own bitterness toward and distrust of men. She has broken part of the family loyalty by being a caring mother to her daughters, even though her own mother wasn't caring with her. If she doesn't resolve more issues with her mother, though, the invisible loyalty will shackle her to a life of bitterness, which she then risks passing on to her daughters.

I explain to Beth that by being bitter, she is actually honoring her loyalty to her mother.

"You've got to be kidding! I don't like her."

"You are following her rules about holding on to bitterness, distrusting men, dragging along with you the emotions of a dead marriage, depriving yourself of inner contentment."

"I don't want to do this," she wails.

"Loyalty is powerful. You can't avoid it; you must honor *some* part of her. But you can choose which part: the negative stuff or any of the good things you got from her."

The only successful way to separate from your parents—because of their destructive influence in your life or because of a closeness that leaves little room for your independent growth—is to go back to them. Go back and make peace with the past. You can't break away from your family loyalty; you can only adjust to it by negotiating (with yourself) how you need to be different from them *as well as* what parts of them you want to maintain.

Changing Negative Loyalty To Positive Loyalty

In *You Can Go Home Again* (W. W. Norton, 1997), Monica McGoldrick says that understanding your connections to your family and family loyalty is a lifetime project. "To create something new, you will have to struggle against the definitions you are given [by family members] so that you can define connectedness in ways that you find meaningful." She wishes her readers the "best of luck with this project of going home again, even though it is never the place you left" (p. 288).

Since you have no choice about being loyal to each parent, it's critical that you make a conscious choice about the ways you remain loyal. First, you need to identify the destructive family rules, behaviors, attributes, and interests—for instance, not trusting men, an out-of-control temper, heavy drinking, bitterness, helplessness. Which ones have you absorbed and repeated?

Then, you need to confront the effect the negative ones have had and still have on your life.

Third, you also need to identify the positive family rules, behaviors, attributes, and interests. This might include being fiscally responsible, openly affectionate, concerned about social injustice. Which ones have you been avoiding or ignoring because you wanted to distance yourself from you parents? Which ones have you embraced, despite your parents?

Fourth, do a self-assessment. Which of the negative family rules do you want to stop?

Fifth, which of the positive ones do you want to maintain and, if you have children, pass on to the next generation?

Finally, it's important to find a way to disengage from the negative loyalty you now have with each parent and express your loyalty to the positive aspects of them. You need to honor that as a gift from them, even if you basically dislike them.

Reflection: Steps For Changing Negative Loyalty To Positive Loyalty

1. Identify your family's destructive rules, behaviors, attributes, and interests. Which ones have you absorbed and repeated?
2. Confront the effect the negative ones have had and still have on your life.
3. Identify your family's positive rules, behaviors, attributes, and interests. Which ones have you avoided? Which ones have you embraced?
4. Choose the negative ones you want to stop.
5. Choose the positive ones you want to maintain and pass on to the next generation.
6. Find a way to disengage from the negative forms of loyalty. Express your loyalty by honoring the positive aspects of your parents.

I suggest to Beth that she take a piece of paper and draw a vertical line down the middle of it to make two columns. On the left side, she's to list all the behaviors and characteristics she admires about her mother. On the right side, she is to list everything she hates.

The following week, Beth brings in a very lopsided list, the hates being five times as long. We talk about her similarities to her mother on each side of the list.

"You can't escape loyalty, but look how you maintain it through the negative similarities. If you were to emphasize the positive similarities, you might not have to hold so tightly to the bitterness and negativism. Using a magic marker, highlight only those characteristics from the positive side that you share with your mom."

Beth picks up the brown marker and grudgingly looks over the list. Then a grin appears on her face. She drops the marker back in the basket and takes out the yellow one. She circles a few items quickly.

When she's finished, Beth's face lights up as she talks about her mother's love of literature. They loved talking about books. She also credits her mother for her musical talent. Beth has sung in the church choir for many years. One of her very few fond memories from childhood is singing with her mother while they washed the dishes together. Her mother was a wonderful cook, and although she never taught Beth how, it is among the rare things they have in common.

Reflection: Identifying Your Positive And Negative Loyalty

Take one sheet of paper for your mother and one for your father and vertically divide each sheet in half. On the left side, write Negative Traits. Under this, for each parent, list those attributes and behaviors that you have gotten that you don't like. Consider "assigned" roles that you incorporated as a child and perpetuated through the family trance, such as *lazy, dumb*. On the right side, write Positive Traits. Under this, list those attributes and behaviors you have gotten from each parent that you value, want to nurture, and pass on if you have children.

Reflection: Removing The Negative Behaviors Or Characteristics

1. On separate index cards, list the behaviors or characteristics you want to eliminate that bind you to your parents through negative loyalty.
2. For each card, draw or cut out pictures, make a collage, or write up a particular incident that represents each behavior.
3. Decide what to do with the cards. You might want to tear them up, burn them, or write them a "eulogy" and then bury them.

Honoring The Positive Loyalty

Once you are clear about the aspects of each parent that you don't want to repeat, and you've identified those that you want to incorporate as part of your life, you need to make a conscious effort to honor them.

Beth now needed to find a way to honor the ways she wanted to maintain her loyalty to her mother.

"I have an idea, but" I hedged, "it might sound really funky, so bear with me. Set up an altar-type area at home for your mother. Use a small unobtrusive corner somewhere. Include in this area anything that represents the positives on your list—a book, musical instrument or record, pie plate, whatever. The idea is to see whether by honoring these positive things—and seeing them every day—you eliminate the need to remain loyal to traits you don't like."

We set an appointment for the following month, but two weeks later Beth left a brief message on my answering machine. "I hate to admit it, but it really seems to be working." She had to cancel her next appointment, so I didn't see her until two months later. The shadowy bitter facial expressions had been replaced by a gentle quietness and her delightful grin.

During the previous two months, Beth had written her mother, who now lives in a nursing home. Beth had no idea about her mother's mental status, but she risked a short, somewhat impersonal note along with a book she thought her mother might enjoy. Two weeks later she received a note, written in a shaky script. Her mother talked about her impressions of the author and the characters, and enclosed a book in exchange. Beth and her mother have continued the book sharing and discussions ever since.

Last week, Beth actually telephoned her mother to pursue a topic from the latest book they've been reading. "It's the first time I've heard her voice in almost a decade. She sounds so different, yet very much the same, if that makes any sense. But don't get too excited," she cautions, reacting to my smile. "This is all superficial stuff. However, I am enjoying the discussions, and I'm curious if it will affect my feelings about her as a mother. I don't know where this is all heading. I'm just letting it flow by itself."

She explains she is still angry at her ex-husband, Carter, but "I haven't had enough time to think much about him lately. Besides, he's bad energy, and I'm infusing myself in such good energy right now. During these past months, I've been exploring my spirituality." (Beth has become involved with a women's group that's studying positive figures such as Mother Earth and female goddesses.)

"I can tell something is changing. I know I'm on a different path than I was before; I have no idea where this is leading me, but it feels right, at least for the time being." Beth doesn't believe she will ever talk to her mother about her childhood—how unfairly she had been treated, how her mother transferred her marital anger to her. Even so, she has mended the cutoff from her mother.

She has found another way to be loyal to her, freeing herself from the negative loyalty of being cold and bitter. Beth can now choose whatever rules she wants to guide her life.

Reflection: Honoring The Positive Aspects Of Loyalty

Here are some ideas for honoring the positive family rules, behaviors, traits, and interests you have inherited from each parent. Use these examples, if they fit, or use them as a jumping-off point to create your own.

Post the Positive

1. On separate brightly colored index cards, list the positives you have gotten from each parent.
2. On each card, draw or cut out pictures, make a collage, or write a story you recall representing the behavior.
2. Post the cards around your home.
3. Make a point of looking at them every day.

Thank You Letter

Write a letter thanking your parent for the gift of the attribute(s). This letter does not need to be sent. The letter can be written even if you are not in contact with the parent, or if the parent is deceased.

Pursue the Trait

Follow up on one of the positive traits you "inherited" from a parent. This is especially important if you've avoided that trait or talent because you have avoided everything about that parent.

Finishing Unfinished Business

Changing loyalty from negative to positive is something you do by yourself. The next step involves your dealing with parents directly (whether or not they are alive and you are in contact with them). You need to finish your unfinished business with them. You may need to get closure on one or more situations from your childhood, and/or you may need to have them treat you differently today.

Beth Erickson, in *Longing for Dad: Father Loss and Its Impact* (Health Communications, 1998), cautions against burying living parents. If your parents are still alive, there may be a chance to connect in some way that gives you some, if not all, of what you need from them, while not acquiescing or giving up yourself.

The point of communicating with parents is to open a dialogue, not a confrontation. The past is over. There is nothing they can do to remove what you have already suffered. However, what you may need today is for them to hear the pain their adult child suffered in her childhood. You may need for them to step outside of who they were back then; from the vantage point of who they are today, you may need them to give you what they couldn't then—an available heart and a good ear.

If you want your parents to treat you differently from when you were a child, you need to teach them how. In order to do that, you first need to prepare yourself. No one has written a book for parenting adult children, so there are no guidelines. You and your parents have to make up your own rules as you go along. I can recommend two guiding principles, however: don't attack and don't defend.

In preparing to talk directly with your parents about important issues, it is crucial that you do it in a way that leaves you feeling good about yourself—regardless of your parents' reactions to what you say. These principles remove the destructive barbs that interfere with genuine communication. It really *is* possible to talk with parents in a calm, non-defensive manner, *regardless of how they respond to you.*

Guidelines For Talking With Parents

Here are four suggestions to get you started.

1. Don't personalize

Most likely, what your parents did or didn't do for you in your childhood had nothing to do with you! Even so, you suffered because of them, and you are entitled to be angry that you didn't get what you needed. It's a parent's responsibility to behave appropriately toward a child and to punish appropriately, not abusively.

You may have been a victim of their own negative loyalty; that is, the baggage they carried from their childhood. Thinking about them as young children who didn't have their needs met might make it easier not to personalize what they did to you.

Some people believe forgiveness is necessary for healing. After years of working with thousands of people, however, I've come to believe that forgiveness is *not* crucial. Some people need to forgive their parents, some don't. What *is* crucial is coming to peace with your anger. Only when you grieve what you didn't get from your parents, only when you find a positive form of loyalty, and let go of the negative loyalty, are you free from your own emotional baggage. And you'll no longer need to personalize your parents' behavior toward you.

2. Who apologizes, and for what?

Can you hear the difference between a parent saying, "I'm sorry for what I did to you," and "I'm sorry for what you suffered as a result of what I did"? It's an important difference. It's nice when parents apologize for their child-rearing mistakes or their abusive behavior, but that doesn't necessarily make an adult child feel her pain has been *heard.* She needs to be comforted by her parents—like her younger self had needed—when she thinks back on having been harmed. She needs a parent to hear the feelings she experienced back then— pain, loneliness, anger, abandonment. Parents who apologize for their behavior are, in fact, removing themselves from the role of comforter; it brings the parents of her childhood up into her present day.

It isn't the present that needs healing, it's the past. Being comforted by your parents, even decades later, can be healing. Many parents miss this distinction. You may need to teach them.

Some parents *are* willing to apologize for their behavior. One developmental task in old age is to reflect on your life, feeling good about your accomplishments and taking responsibility for your errors. This may be the time for your parents to make peace within themselves, which means owning up to their mistakes with you. This often is a time of softening, so whereas they may have been cruel or self-centered before, they may be more open to hearing you now.

You are lucky if your mom and dad (separately) are able to go the first step and acknowledge: "I made some bad mistakes, and I accept responsibility for them. I wish I had done things differently." You are even more fortunate if your parents can hear *the effect* their behaviors had on you. If your parents can't, though, don't be surprised if their apology doesn't make you feel any better. That's because what they're doing is for *their* development and peace of mind, not necessarily *yours*.

Some parents refuse to take any responsibility—period. If so, then it's important for you to say what you need to say, holding on to your reality of what happened. Don't worry if they say you've distorted the facts. What you *feel* about the past, regardless of the facts, has more bearing at this stage of talking with them. If they won't accept responsibility, don't argue with them. Keep holding your own. That in itself may help you get some closure and peace of mind.

After several years of therapy, Starr decided to confront her father with his having sexually abused her. She was still in touch with both parents, but this was a major issue that silently loomed between her and her father. Her father denied the abuse. He wasn't particularly angry at her accusation; he just insisted he didn't do it.

After the confrontation, Starr reported, "I'm fine. *I* know it happened, that's what's important. I would feel closer to him if he had [confessed], but I feel 50 pounds lighter just having told him, having it out in the open. I may or may not ever need to raise it again. It'll be easier to spend time with him now, although it might be harder for him. That's his problem."

Some parents accept responsibility for their behavior but not for the effect it has had on your life. They may say, "I've made mistakes, but it's up to you now to change your life." That's true. Unfortunately, they aren't being comforting parents to the younger you left inside.

3. Anticipate resistance to change

Think about two people on a seesaw. In order to have the best ride, they need to find the balance point on the board. If one person moves up or back, changing the balance, the other *has* to move in order to rebalance the board. Or they have to stop seesawing altogether.

Using the seesaw image, prepare yourself for your parents' reaction to your shifting the way you relate to them. The one who is most uncomfortable with the relationship is the one who will shift first. This usually is the adult child. If the parents want to continue relating to that child, who has changed the balance, then they are forced to move. Since the parents are not asking for change, they may resist it and attempt to return to the status quo, trying to regain the old balance.

If you are prepared with this understanding of change and resistance to it, dealing with your parents may be less frustrating. You will anticipate their blocking your efforts, their pulling back toward the status quo. If it's important to establish a different type of relationship with them, be ready to hold firm as they resist your first move. What you do in your second and third moves is where the real change can occur.

Using a typical, yet generic, example, let's see how this works. An adult child and her father are in a discussion. He starts yelling—either at her or just because of his energetic response to the topic.

First Move

Adult Child: "Dad, please don't yell; it scares me." [Having never mentioned this before, she initiates the change.]

Father: "How dare you talk to me like that?" [He is resisting change. By doing what he always does, using intimidation, he expects she will back off and respond as she always does. This keeps the status quo.}

Second Move

Adult Child: "I'd like to hear what you are saying to me, but I can't if you are yelling." [She doesn't have to get stopped by the resistance; she can hold her ground.]

Father: "Don't you dare talk back to me." [He repeats his resistance, trying to maintain their communication status quo. He may yell louder, try to hit her, swear at her, or just swear in general. He also may withdraw and walk away, become pathetic, or berate himself for being a lousy father.]

Third Move

Adult Child: "I don't want you yelling at me, so I'm going for a walk (or home). I'll be back in 10 or 15 minutes (or tomorrow); maybe we can talk better then." [This is done without anger or rancor in her voice. The message is clear. She's taking the initiative to change the way they relate.]

Father: [Screaming} "Fine, and don't ever step foot in this house again!"

Fourth Move

Adult Child: "Goodbye, Dad. See you later." [Ignoring his threat, she plans to resume contact with him, as normal, talking to him the next time *as if this had never happened!* Yet, she holds on to her new resolve of not talking with him if he yells at her.]

The daughter has made her changing moves and can see that the effect has caused her father to thrash around trying to reassert the old pattern of relating. If she keeps holding him to the new rules, they both gain—only he doesn't know that just yet.

Be prepared; holding to your planned change is often difficult in the face of a resistant parent. In fact, the more intimidating or guilt-inducing the parent, the more difficult it is to hold your ground without showing anger or backing down. However, if your parent has any desire for contact with you, it probably won't cause a fatal cutoff. It may take a number of repetitions, though, before he learns the new rules of relating to you.

1. Know what you want

This fourth guideline is the most crucial one. If you don't know what you want out of talking with your parents, you may not get it. Or you won't know if you've gotten it. Ask yourself: What do I want from talking with Mom? From Dad? Do I want them to treat me as an adult? Do I want to understand why certain things happened in the family when I was growing up? Or, do I just want them to stop complaining about me and my lifestyle? Be clear with yourself: Do you want to focus on the past, on your current situation, or both?

Beth was able to go home again (by mail and telephone) as an unshackled adult child. She took charge of changing the relationship she had with her mother. She didn't want to deal with the past, but she wanted a way for them to connect in the present. She limited herself to their common interest—reading. If her mother raised other topics, Beth gave a noncommittal response and returned to safe ground. Beth set new ground rules, and her mother accepted them. By changing her own behavior, she opened the possibility of getting more from her mother. Soon the two women were able to stretch the areas of their communication.

Teaching Them To Treat You Differently

What looks like parental "resistance" to treating you differently may actually be a lack of know-how. You need to teach them, and you need to give them space to grieve their obsolescence, the loss of their role as parents to you as a child. In addition, they may need to grieve what they lose by your being single (see Chapter 10).

Most parents need some assistance in learning how to relate to their children as adults. It is unrealistic to expect them to suddenly change from seeing you as their child to treating you with the same deference they do other adults.

While many parents have difficulty with this transition with all of their children, Always Single women often feel parents treat them as if they are younger than their married siblings, regardless of the children's birth order. As many women have said, "You just aren't seen as grown up until you have a husband."

You can force your family to treat you as an adult in specific ways, however. Remember the story of my piano (see Chapter 2)? By not speaking up, I colluded with everyone in saying, "Karen cannot have the piano until she is married." It is up to *you* to speak up!

Do you collude with your family's not treating you as grown up? Over the years, I have asked my midlife graduate students if they have ever had the family over for a holiday dinner. Almost unanimously, married women and men and Single Again mothers respond affirmatively. Always Singles are usually surprised at the idea. It's as if they have been in a trance that says holidays must be celebrated at the home of their parents or married siblings.

Child-free Single Agains may have had the family over when they were married, but many of them say not since their divorce. When I ask why family dinners are hosted by marrieds, the answers come quickly—perhaps too quickly: "It's too difficult to bring the whole family to my house." "My home isn't big enough."

Yet, when they think more objectively about it, these single women realize there would be no difference if their sister and brother brought the kids to their parents' home or to their own. One woman seemed quite taken with the discussion. After a long silence, she said, "I just never thought about it."

Another question I ask my students is: "How many Always Singles have ever cooked a whole turkey?" Not that cooking a turkey is a rite of passage, but not having done it often leaves a person feeling less adult. Maybe it's a carry-over from childhood, when mother cooked and the children just showed up, ate, and cleared the table.

Three Teaching Methods

Basically, you have three ways to choose from in teaching your parents how to treat you as an adult. You can do it directly, indirectly, or by letter. Whichever way you choose, you need to be clear about your goals. Further, don't act out of anger and, whenever possible, use humor.

The Direct Method

In order for the direct method to be successful, you need to do your homework. First, you have to *collect your data*. What are the comments or behaviors from each family member that bother you the most? It may be the things they do, the words they use, or the ideas they have about you and your life. Rather than just being annoyed, write down their comments. This gives you time to think about how you want to respond. An off-the-cuff retort, made in anger, is rarely heard and, consequently, is not effective in making a change.

Next, you need to *categorize and prioritize* your complaints. Don't overload your family with too much at once. Look over your list of complaints for each family member. See if the items can be grouped in a few categories. For instance, even though you're 38 years old and own your own home, your mom still tells you to drive safely, not to stay out too late, and to be careful about the men you are meeting. These comments may all be grouped under her lack of trust in your decision making and your inability to take care of yourself.

Comments about not keeping your house clean, or not wearing the right makeup or clothes, may be grouped under her not respecting how you are different from her. Once you have categorized the complaints, prioritize them, and select the category that bothers you most. If several bother you, pick any one for starters.

Plan your approach, *strategize*. Decide how to talk to each person in a non-inflammatory way; never try to talk seriously when the person is angry or busy. Find a quiet time, or set a date specifically to talk about "something important to me." Think about something in the person's life that will help him or her connect with your feelings.

Margaret, whom we met in Chapter 1, tells this story.

"One day I asked Mom if she would meet me for lunch. I said I wanted to talk about something important. We chatted for a while before I got up the courage to broach the subject.

"I can't remember exactly what I said, but it went something like this. 'I appreciate your willingness to talk with me about something that's important to me. Remember you told me you used to feel criticized every time your mother visited you? She wasn't respecting the way your were living your life. She may have thought she was being helpful, but you only felt it as a criticism.

"'Well, thank goodness you're different with me than she was with you. Yet, there is one similarity. It really bothers me when you make comments that sound like you don't respect our differences. You often say if I were married, I'd keep a cleaner house, or I'd dress better. I hope you can trust that I have learned how to take care of myself, even if it is in a way that is different from you.

"'You didn't feel that talking with your mother would help. I do hope our talking about this will help, that you will want to respect my feelings. When you make these comments, it makes me feel like a child, and it also makes me angry. I suspect you have never thought about how it feels to me when you say these things. I also know you don't mean to make me angry about this.'"

Margaret catches her breath and sighs, as if she has just had the conversation with her mother, not just repeated it. "I then talked about how I could help her catch herself so she didn't keep doing it. We decided to use a silly catchword each time one of us heard her say any of the bothersome comments. We chose pea soup, a food she *hates*. So, she is certain to laugh if I say it, rather than feel criticized."

The Indirect Method

Sometimes, an indirect means of communicating can be more useful—especially if it is well targeted and done humorously. I loved my father and knew he loved me, but he just couldn't stop treating me like a child. Telling him directly when I didn't like something he said or did proved useless. It took me until my early 30s to figure out a formula for not feeling like a child with him.

Ever since my college days, my father would slip me money on my visits home. When I was in my early 20s, I loved it. In my late 20s, I didn't want to make him feel bad by telling him I felt uncomfortable taking it. By the time I had reached my 30s, I found it insulting, even though I knew my father respected me as an adult and as a professional. I knew there was nothing belittling in his action; yet it still made me feel small, helpless, and needy. I knew his giving me money was his way of showing he loved me, as well as adhering to his socialization that fathers take care of their daughters until they get married and a husband takes over the job. Regardless, I wanted him to stop. I tried getting angry, sending it back, talking to him about it. Nothing worked.

Finally, I got smart. If I couldn't change his cultural upbringing, I could change the *meaning* of his action. So, whenever he visited me, I slipped *him* money. Not only did we have a delightful game, it changed how I felt. I was participating as an adult in the very same game I used to participate in as a child.

The Letter Method

When there is hostility, on your part or your parents', you may need some distance as you teach them what you need. Communicating initially by letter provides a precautionary safety net. You can write and rewrite your letter until you say exactly what you want. You can edit out sarcasm, defensiveness, pandering.

The recipient of the letter wins too by being able to react without worrying about the sender witnessing their reaction. With a letter, the receiver may hear different intentions on each successive reading. After a range of reactions, the receiver can write and rewrite a well-considered response.

In *Longing for Dad* (Health Communication, 1998), Beth Erickson quoted a letter written from a woman to her father that provides a model for clearing up old business with a parent (pp. 200–201). The woman told her parents the reason she was writing was to ask them for help in getting her life in order. She affirmed her love for them. She clarified that the intention of her letter was to improve her relationship with them, not to hurt them. The tone of her letter was empathic, not condemnatory. While some might feel such a letter would have to be confrontational, her request actually gave her parents the opportunity to parent her in the present, to make up for their shortcomings when she was a child. It opened, not closed, a dialogue between the adult daughter and her parents.

She did not blame them or accuse them of anything, but she did ask them to take responsibility for their actions when she was a child. She articulated what she wanted and needed from them and made concrete suggestions. (For more ideas about using letters in dealing with your parents, see Terry Vance's *Letters Home* [Pantheon, 1998.])

Whether you are able to talk with your parents directly or through letter writing, it's important to settle and then bury the unfinished business with them. If you don't, the issues hang around forever, even in disguise. They interfere with your adult relationships and, if you have children, get passed on to another generation. If you are having difficulty doing this, consider using a professional therapist. To complete the task of making peace with your parents, you need to lighten your suitcase of emotional baggage.

Self-Assessment

The eighth task, Making Peace with Your Parents, involves four key issues. Look them over to see how you are doing in each one.

Identifying Your Family Rules And Loyalty Style

Recognizing Your Family Loyalty

___identify your style of negative loyalty
___identify your style of positive loyalty
___remove your negative loyalty
___honor your positive loyalty

Identifying Your Unfinished Business

___establish your guidelines for talking with parents
___don't personalize
___pay attention to the apology
___anticipate resistance to change

Teaching Your Parents To Treat You Differently

___use the direct method
___use the indirect method
___use the letter-writing method

For any category that you are satisfied with, give yourself a "star," either figuratively or literally. For any that you still need to work on, think about what needs to be added or changed in order for it to be satisfactory. Then, write your ideas for that category.

If you are stuck, talk with friends or family to see how they handle that task. If you are still stuck after that, consider reading a self-help book, taking a course that deals with the topic, or talking with a professional psychotherapist or pastoral counselor who specializes in family relationships.

12

Preparing For Old Age

Lifestyle, friends and family, men, work, money—these are important issues to look at in planning ahead, in preparing for old age, the ninth task.

We talk about old age as if we know what it means, as if we know when we reach it. For most people, old age is simply . . . later! We live in a world that is terrified of growing old. Being young and vital is a national obsession. Even with the number of books, seminars, and television shows on aging, the topic has still not mobilized more respect and value toward old people.

But I'm not interested in identifying a specific number for the onset of old age. My goal in this chapter is to discuss the task of preparing for this life stage. My good friend Sharon has done just that.

Wearing Purple

It's New Year's Eve. We're sitting in Sharon's living room overlooking the bay. I ask, "Do you make resolutions?"

"I don't call them resolutions, but I do think about what I want to focus on for the coming year."

At 60, Sharon is a proud single mother whose one grown son has an exciting career and is close to both her and his father. She is very successful at work and has moved up the career ladder. A few years ago, she sold her home in a big city and resettled in a coastal town where she could have a quieter life. She bought a great house; she's willed it to her son (which means she has a will), and she has images of (hopefully) future grandchildren playing here.

Her answering machine tells you she's out watching the water. That's only partly true. Some of the time she's weaving baskets, meeting with her women's investment group, talking with good friends, like tonight. Our conversation flows easily.

"I need to decide where men fit into my life now," Sharon muses. "After my divorce, I had no time for a serious relationship, I was so busy just trying to make a life for my son. Since then, I've had lovers, but no serious relationship.

I would like a man, but I need to decide how much I should invest in thinking about that.

"The other thing I need to think about this year is if I want to retire. I'm not sure I'll have enough money; besides, I would really miss working. Do I want to see if my company will let me stay part time? Or do I want something entirely different? I'm meeting with my financial planner next month to see what I can do to expand my financial options."

Like Sharon, all women need to address the issues of aging. Gloria Steinem, in an interview in the May-June 1999 issue of *Modern Maturity,* the magazine of the American Association of Retired Persons, suggests three alternatives for thinking about yourself as old. In the first, you can "go along with society's vision of aging and become *an older woman of a conventional sort*" (emphasis added). This, presumably, is the image of the gracious former First Lady, Barbara Bush.

The second alternative is to "defy society's idea of aging by remaining *a younger woman of a conventional sort*" (again, emphasis added). You know this woman; she is the one who spends lots of hours and money on makeup and reconstructive cosmetic surgery to remove all signs of her body's aging. The end result is that while each piece of her looks young, she's still an old woman packaged in her age-defying body.

The third alternative for thinking about yourself as an old woman is "refusing to honor others' expectations" of who you should be. However, Steinem says, finding your own image doesn't come easily. For example, she had intended to ignore her own aging. "I definitely greeted [my 50s] with defiance." She assumed she would "dress the same way and act the same way," as she always had, and if people didn't like it, too bad.

Somewhere along that decade, she realized that being who she had been before was not progress. That was only "staying the person you were. Stasis is never growth. It's preferable to adapting to someone's idea of what you should be, but it's a sorry alternative to using your age and experience to move on to something else.

"As you age," Steinem continues, "there is a belated feeling of being less dependent on the approval of others, and therefore [a willingness] to push the boundaries. . . . Today, I'm much more likely to say what I think and not worry about hurting somebody's feelings" (pp. 52–53).

That's the premise too of a poem by Jenny Joseph, "When I Am Old I Shall Wear Purple" (the title Sandra Martz chose for her edited poetry collection published by Papier-Mâché Press in 1987). Older women have the freedom to be and do whatever they choose, whether that's a recluse or a purple-bedecked outlandish female. Midlife women have paid their dues of propriety and of following the rules; now they can choose for themselves who they want to be and how they want to behave.

Compare Steinem's and Joseph's attitude about being an older single woman with Lila's. A Single Again woman in her mid-60s, Lila is unhappy being single, so it's no surprise that she's doubly unhappy being an aging single. When asked what it's like for her, she almost literally cringes, "I don't want to think about it!" Her voice cracks with tangible fear.

When I press further, asking Lila why, it's even harder to get her to talk about why she can't talk about it. "I just don't want to." Since her divorce left her financially secure, it appears her reaction is about being "alone and old."

Lila's reaction may be more extreme than how most other single women would react, or she might just be more obvious about her fear. Many single women do fear aging by themselves. In talking with so many single women over the years, I've noticed that the word they usually associate with old is "alone." The mantra is, "I don't want to be old and alone." But do these two words necessarily have to go together? Does a single woman have to grow old alone?

Perhaps Lila would be less fearful of being alone if years ago she had begun thinking about being a woman in her mid-60s one day. If she had paid more attention to improving her relationships with her children, her friends, and her siblings, she wouldn't feel alone now—with or without a husband.

Personal Needs

Single midlife women should consider two basic needs—nurturance and connection—as they prepare for their next life stage, aging. Improving relationships with the important people who will be with you in old age will soften the aloneness.

Most studies on aging recognize three levels of personal needs: concrete needs, socialization, and emotional needs. Each need is met by a different set of people. For their concrete or tangible needs, the elderly tend to turn to their children. They turn to their friends for socialization. And for their emotional needs, they turn to their siblings.

Preparing For Old Age—Your Children

Research on the aged suggests that old people turn to their children for help with such concrete needs as rides to the doctor, medical problems, grocery shopping, financial decisions. It can be mutually rewarding for parents, who gave lovingly to you, to accept the turnaround of you, the adult child, giving back to them. On the other hand, if parent and child were never close, when that parent becomes old and needy, it can be difficult for both. The parent needs the help, but the adult child resents having to give what she never received.

Before you reach the point of being so physically or emotionally dependent on your children, think about what type of relationship you would like to have with them, now and later. You can amend the slogan "It's never too late to have a happy childhood" to "It's never too late to have a good relationship with your adult child."

In Chapter 11, you, the adult child, considered making peace with your parents. Now, in thinking about your old age, you are the parent to your adult children. You can make amends to them in a way you might have wished your parents had with you. By improving this relationship, you are not only preparing for your old age, you are freeing your children from any negative loyalty bind they may have with you.

When you are in the parent rather than the adult child role, you, as mother, are the one who initiates change and pushes for an improved relationship. Three of the four guidelines for teaching your parents to treat you as an adult (as described in Chapter 11) can now be used to finish unfinished business with your children.

1. Take responsibility for what you did or didn't do to your children. Be sure to take responsibility for the effect of your behaviors on them. While you may want to explain yourself, don't be surprised if they are less interested in your explanation than in hearing you acknowledge the pain you caused them.

2. Anticipate their resistance to change. They may have held a grudge against you for years. They may not be so ready to let go. You may find yourself being pulled back into old behaviors you don't like. Hold firm, remembering the importance of your second and third moves. (You may want to reread this section in Chapter 10.)

3. Know what you want for your improved relationship. Having an end picture may make it easier to keep your eye on your goal and not get sidetracked by your child's attempts to block your change. Do you want to be able to talk about the past? Do you want more contact with your grandchildren? Do you want to be able to share more of your current lives with each other?

The same three methods for achieving this with your parents are applicable, now, with your adult children: deal with them directly, indirectly, or by letter. If none of these methods proves rewarding, consider the professional assistance of a family therapist. Don't give up too soon!

There is yet a fourth way to prepare for thinking about your old age with your children. Typically, adult children visit at their parents' home. However, when you get older, retire, and have more free time, will you wait for them to come to you or will you go to them?

My mother and father, for example, had two different models from their parents. My mother's mother proudly stated: "I want a good relationship with my daughter, so I'll never intrude. I'll visit only when invited." My mother, now old herself, repeats her mother's words with great pride and independence.

My father's father had an entirely different orientation. His six children lived across the country. He spent his widowed years visiting each one, sometimes up to a month at a time. He'd call and ask, "When do you want me?" If my father had survived my mother, I'm sure that would have been his approach. I'll be curious how my brothers and I each deal with this as we get old.

You don't have to wait, though. You can set the stage now for what you want. If you want to be going to your children's homes, then you can start that now. You can suggest celebrating holidays at their homes, perhaps rotating homes. You can schedule visits with them, for no particular reason. You can begin to find your place in their homes now so you'll feel comfortable and familiar visiting as you age.

Think about the overt and covert messages you've gotten over the years from your parents about adult children's responsibility to their aging parents. How do you imagine that will influence your attitude toward relying on your children when you are old? Do you like your parents' role model, or would you prefer to do something different? You may relate quite differently to each of your children, so you might envision various scenarios with each in your older years. What are their expectations? This may be a good time to start a dialogue with your children.

When you don't have children of your own, knowing that old people look to their children to meet their concrete needs is *not* enough reason to decide to have a child! But if you don't have a child, it raises a good question: Who *will* you look to for support in your old age?

Saying, "No one; I can handle it myself," discounts the reality of needing caring people around to assist you when you're old. Single women without children, therefore, may intentionally nurture friendships with their nieces, nephews, or other young people. This is not self-serving. It is a reciprocal relationship that pays off royally now and also has the potential for long-term benefits for each of you.

If you don't get along with your siblings, access to their children may be difficult. You may need to improve your relationship with them first (see the section below titled "Olive Branches"), or you may just need to be more creative. You can start now to build a relationship with your sibling's children through sending cards and/or "letters" recorded on cassette tapes. You can maintain a one-sided friendship until your sibling softens with age or the child is old enough to respond to you directly.

If you don't have siblings; if your siblings don't have children; if you don't happen to like your siblings' children; or if you can't get around siblings who block your relationships with their children, you can still find ways to develop a rapport with a special child. You might take in a foster child. You might get better acquainted with your godchild (if you have one). Or you might "adopt" a niece or nephew by befriending a close friend's son or daughter.

Preparing For Old Age: Your Friends

When you are old, your social network narrows as your friends die, become more self-absorbed with their medical problems, or become less mentally competent. Watching your friends decline can be depressing and can affect your own attitude about aging.

Edith recalls the last two decades in the life of her mother, a woman who died at 93. "She was miserable. Her large network of friends diminished in size, and after my father died, Mom became reclusive. She still had a few friends, but she didn't like them. I used to ask her, 'How can you not like your friends? If they're your friends, you like them, right?' She would get indignant, as if I were really stupid. She'd start a litany of complaints about the three women she still talked to each week.

"It was curious, and I assumed she was just being cranky. Until I went to lunch one day with Mom and two of these friends. I had known them my whole life and was really quite fond of them. But over lunch, I saw what my mother was talking about. They were totally wrapped up in themselves and their illnesses. They could not stay involved in a conversation for more than a few paragraphs before they had a complaint about a person, referred to their physical ailments, or were nasty to my mother.

"Later, I apologized to my mother. It got me really worried, though, about myself. Would I be like that when I got old? Worse, would my friends? Would I lose them to crankiness and nastiness? I never could have imagined that these two women who used to be so bright, and funny, and cared so much about me would have turned into boring, self-absorbed, unpleasant old ladies."

You have no assurance of what will happen to your friends as they age. What you can do now, though, in preparation for old age, is pay close attention to maintaining or increasing your social network, nurturing and taking good care of your friendships. This may be a critical factor in your making a healthy adjustment to old age.

Many midlife women *have* begun thinking about their friends and friendships in their old age. "When I'm old," says my 62-year-old friend Zina, "I want to get a group of friends to move into the same apartment building. We'll share the cost of hiring a driver, so we won't have to worry about having a car. We'll share the cost of hiring a cook who will make dinners for us, and we'll rotate eating in each one's home."

My friend Carol is also 62. She has a fantasy "for when I'm old" which includes buying a big house together with her friends. She hasn't yet figured out the details, such as which friends she wants to live with and in which city the house will be.

Mallory, a 52-year-old friend, has a different idea. "When I'm old, I want my friends to all have a second home in different parts of the country, or even in different countries. That way we can spend our old age traveling around visiting each other. Me, I want a villa in Italy. I hope someone picks the Northern California coast and someone else picks the mountains. That way, I'll be able to visit the ocean and continue horseback riding in the mountains."

Whether these are realistic plans or just fantasies doesn't matter. What these women are doing is not only talking about their future living situation, but also about bringing their good friends with them into old age.

This new idea—thinking about friendships in old age—is also contributing to the number of senior communities for the well and healthy that are popping up around the country. They offer a full range of activities and a social life inside their borders. By moving in when they are well, single and married women and men are establishing new friendships among their neighbors, who will be close by as they age.

Nursing homes for people who cannot take care of themselves used to be the sole option for the elderly. But since the elderly are living longer and leading fuller lives, different levels of housing have evolved. Between the independent living and nursing homes are the assisted living environments for those who need some help with their basic daily needs, but who can still take an active part in life.

In her *Modern Maturity* interview, Gloria Steinem spoke of a collective-living group called The Last Perch whose "philosophy was that if each of them had one remaining faculty, then together they had all five." Now, that's friendship! And I've heard several women quip, "When I'm old and infirm, I want to move into the same nursing home with my friends" (pp. 52–53). That, perhaps, may be the best insurance policy against being old and alone.

Developing Younger Friendships

Developing relationships with friends who are much younger than you is another way to build a support system for your older years. Donna, a woman whose adult life has been spent mostly overseas, intuitively understood that. "Since coming back to live in the States, one of the things I'm consciously doing is cultivating friendships with young people. Even at my age [58], I've become aware that my contemporaries are dropping. This way, as my same-age friends die or become infirm, I will have friendships that can continue."

There's nothing crass about intentionally seeking out younger people to be a part of your life. If it's a true friendship, you'll both gain from it now, and if you're lucky (there are no guarantees), you'll both reap the rewards later.

Preparing For Old Age: Your Siblings

Most people are aware of the importance of children and friends in the lives of the elderly. What may *not* be as well known is the importance of siblings in meeting the psychological and emotional needs of the elderly. About 95 percent of Americans have at least one birth sibling. This relationship is usually the longest one you'll ever have. Parents most often die before their children; spouses and friends come later in your life. And, unlike with them, you can't divorce your siblings.

Sibling relationships can be highly complex and emotionally charged. Their quality is not static; they may weave in and out of your life in varying degrees of intensity, depending on your age and your life situation.

Think of the sibling relationship as an hourglass. The top of the hourglass is bigger because you have much more contact with each other in childhood. The hourglass progressively narrows as you move into your young adulthood, and somewhere around midlife it begins to broaden again. As research indicates, the hourglass returns to its largest size in old age, when you have increasingly more interaction with your siblings.

Midlife Adulthood

As your parents get older, get sick, or die, you and your siblings may have to deal more with each other. The old jealousies or other unfinished business with them may indirectly resurface around the task of making decisions for or about your parents. Your frozen images of your siblings as bossy, manipulative, shirking their chores, for instance, get transferred to this new task.

The ways in which you differ in helping your parents may reflect your childhood style of arguing: pitting one sib against another, going behind the other's back, passive-aggressively "giving up." The questions about allegiances may be the same as back then: who sides with which parent, who feels left out or favored, who is caught between your parents or between one parent and a sibling?

Among the myriad reasons why the unfinished business from childhood resurfaces is that by fighting with each other, keeping the focus on your siblings, you all avoid the reality of your parents' aging (and your own). You avoid any grief or guilt you have about your parents. You don't have to ask yourself hard questions: Did you get what you needed from your parents? What unfinished business do you still have with them? Have you done enough for them now?

Along with this suitcase of old feelings are current ones. Fighting with your siblings can deflect you from feelings of inadequacy and helplessness because you cannot cure your parents or relieve their pain.

Your own midlife and your parents' aging bring you face to face with your mortality. Preparing for or dealing with the loss of your parents often raises feelings about your becoming an "adult orphan," the older generation. You have to confront (or avoid confronting) how life is running out on you. You look into the mirror and wonder, Who is that old woman?

Old Age

If you don't have a good relationship with your siblings, take heart. Researcher Victor Cicerrelli confirms that the hourglass really does return to its fullest in old age as your siblings assume more importance in your life. By age 65, more than one-half of people with siblings talk to or see them at least once a week. Many even move so they can live closer to each other in their declining years.

While the old rivalries may still be there, they have softened or are just avoided. No matter how intense the hostility during childhood or the middle adult years, by old age, only 3 percent of siblings cut themselves off from each other, that is, go through their last years without any contact with their sisters and brothers.

Perhaps the most important thing siblings provide for each other in old age is the validation that they once had been young and vital. They are the only ones who know that you used to be skinny; they are the only ones who remember the home run you hit, or the cigarettes you used to sneak in the garage.

When retelling these exploits, you *are* that 11-year-old, not the wrinkled face in the mirror. In old age, siblings provide a continuity of your family history, the scrapbook of family stories. They are the only ones who can laugh—60 or 80 years later—at the mere mention of Uncle Ruby, shorthand for the longer story of how every Passover he spilled red wine on the white tablecloth.

Switching Shoes: Harry And Mary

With rare exceptions, siblings need each other in old age. If you don't have a good relationship now, you may want to think about how to change that, how to prepare for a time when you *will* want to get along with your siblings. To do that, you need to understand the ingredients that are causing tensions today and how they have wended their way from childhood through the decades, still needling you. You need to understand this from your perspective and from your siblings' perspective too.

A successful businessman in his late 50s, Harry is a married man with three children. His father died 10 years ago, and he now lives several hours away from his mother. Harry is a caring son, calling his mother weekly and visiting every other month. His sister, Mary, is six years younger, divorced, and raising two children while working as a secretary in a large architectural firm. She lives 15 minutes away from their mother.

"I don't understand why Mary is always so angry at me. No matter what I do for Mom or her, she's nasty to me. Now she won't even talk to me."

It wasn't always like this. As a child, Mary adored her older brother. She didn't really mind that he was the family prince (first son, smart, good-looking) because he let her tag along with him and his friends.

When he left for college, though, Mary felt totally abandoned. He was so much a part of her life, and then he was gone. And what was worse, he didn't even notice her pain. He never wrote her, and when he came home, he spent little time with her. She was no longer special to him. Without his loving attention, she was left with her built-up resentment that he was the family favorite.

Now, 40 years later, that resentment has only deepened as Mary endures her mother's constant praise for Harry. She is the one there every day taking care of her mother's needs, even while working full time and caring for her children. She is the one making the everyday decisions for her mother. Yet, her mother will call Harry to see what he thinks of Mary's decisions. "I do all the work, and Harry gets all the glory! I feel undermined and totally unappreciated."

While angry at her mother, Mary is more angry about Harry's not noticing. They are at an impasse. From inside Harry's shoes, he views Mary's anger as irrational. He cares about Mary and is hurt that regardless of how much he does for her, she is mean to him and now totally avoids him. His self-image is frozen as the helpful big brother; she is the one who has changed, from loving to nasty.

From inside Mary's shoes, she resents Harry's being idolized by their mother and his insensitivity to her position. His leaving her with the primary burden of caring for their mother (without appreciating her efforts and sacrifice) re-creates for Mary his abandoning her when he went off to college. Her frozen image of Harry is as the adored son she plays second fiddle to.

If only they could switch shoes, viewing the situation from the other's perspective, they would realize how the issues from childhood have permeated their adult lives. Without that, they might move into their old age carrying their resentment. If nothing changes, they are at risk of being in the 3 percent of siblings who are cut off from each other.

Olive Branches

Sometimes, it's not too late. Harry and Mary were lucky. Neither of them asked for help, but when their mother had a stroke, the hospital social worker brought them together to plan her discharge. Through the therapist's skill, brother and sister heard each other's complaints. They had a chance to air their perspectives and confront their unfinished business.

Harry *had* valued Mary's efforts with their mother; he just assumed she knew that. It never occurred to him to tell her. Something as simple as that began the shift that resulted in better coordination around taking care of their mother and more openness and caring between them.

I was once asked to consult at a nursing home with two sisters, 90 and 91 years old. They were still squabbling about which one their mother had loved more, and the wrongs they did to each other back in elementary school. Their adult children (some of them grandparents themselves) requested the consultation because they wanted their mothers to be able to die in peace, caring about each other.

After I was with them just a short time, it became clear: they *did* care about each other—very much. As the sole survivors of their family, they were fighting as a way of holding on to their history, to keep their mother alive. Arguing, for them, *was* caring. If they had been younger, I might have helped them find a less inflammatory way of showing their connection and affection.

You *are* younger; you've got the time to think ahead. Picture yourself in your 70s, 80s, 90s. What type of relationship do you hope to have with your siblings? You may have already tried offering an olive branch, only to have had it refused. If so, or if you have turned down a branch, try this exercise.

Imagine switching shoes with your siblings. See if, *from their perspective,* you can figure how you have hurt, abandoned, or angered them. If you can see from inside their shoes, you may get ideas about a different type of branch.

Olive branches come in a variety of shapes. (Some of them may also work well for improving relationships with your children and your friends.) If you have several siblings, the same method may not work for each. Think about what you know of each sibling and choose a method that has the best chance of being accepted.

Letter Writing

If there is friction, or if you don't believe talking will work, start by writing a letter. Use the same guidelines as suggested for making peace with your parents (Chapter 11): don't attack, don't defend. For example, you might start your letter by stating that you miss being able to talk and be together. How you want to feel closer, or how you hate the silence or hostility between you two. You might explain that soon you'll be the only remaining family members, or that you already are adult orphans, and, therefore, you need each other.

Then, you might spell out the problems, making it clear this is your perspective alone, and you want to hear theirs. If you can tolerate it, ask to hear their perspective first, *before* giving yours. For example, "I'd appreciate your helping me understand if I have done anything to upset you. I feel a coldness between us that I hate. You're very important to me, so I want us to try fixing this. Why don't you tell me your version of the problem?"

You rarely absorb what the other person says until you feel you are understood. Unfortunately, though, someone must always go second.

Be sure to explain you are not attacking your sibling, and you don't mean to be defensive. Acknowledge that putting the two perspectives together might give you both a fuller picture of how the tensions got started, what kept them fueled, and what has prevented a resolution. You might end your letter by asking for a written response. Suggest that the emotional distance of a letter may allow for a better dialogue in which each of you can hear the other better.

If you get a response, write back, being sure to give it the same consideration as your first letter. Keep the letters going back and forth, always talking in terms of wanting to learn more about each other's perspective.

Talking In Person

Another option in offering an olive branch is to invite your sibling (if local) to lunch to specifically discuss how to improve your relationship. This can work if the tension isn't so raw. Having some guidelines in advance, though, may ensure a more productive dialogue. Setting ground rules can be done by letter, by phone, or in person. They might include:

- One person talks at a time.
- You each repeat back what you hear to make sure you are hearing correctly.
- Don't speak for someone who isn't present.
- Agree in advance what topics to talk about and which toxic ones to avoid.
- Don't try to cover too much in one meeting. If it goes well, you can always meet again.

It's a good idea to meet on neutral territory, with no other family member present: a restaurant, a museum lobby, a park. Turn off your cell phones and pagers. Allow yourselves time (don't squeeze this in between other obligations). Or agree in advance on a time frame: "Let's meet between 1 and 3." Guidelines assure a safe structure before walking into a scary arena.

If your sibling lives out of town, you might suggest meeting halfway for a day or a weekend. Plan to do things you both enjoy, such as going to the theater, shopping. Don't mix the talking with the fun time; set aside specific time (or several times) for talking and then go have fun again.

Therapy Consultation

If the tension is too high for letter writing or meeting in person, you might invite your sibling to attend a therapy session with you. A family therapist often can be helpful in clarifying your different versions of past events, unraveling old rivalries, and putting the unresolved "stuff" to rest. This might be a one-time consultation or a few sessions focused specifically on improving your relationship.

As a result of the increased interest in sibling relationships, a few years ago I started offering "Unique Retreats for Siblings." This is a weekend held in the countryside that combines workshops to address the problems, along with a massage and a physical activity, such as horseback riding, hiking, or skiing. These retreats—for all siblings or just sisters—are an opportunity to untangle the old relationships while reestablishing a new one with the people who have known you the longest and who will go into old age with you.

Ideas For Improving Your Midlife Sibling Relationship

1. Letter writing
2. Talking on neutral territory
3. Weekend get-together combining talking and doing
4. Therapy consultation
5. Weekend retreat

Add your own ideas

6._____
7._____

Caution! Some siblings are so damaged from the pain of growing up in their family that reconnection is not possible or even desirable. Don't give up too soon, but don't hold on to an abusive situation. Sometimes, though, it is difficult to know the difference. For instance, if you were physically or sexually abused by a sibling (or you were the abuser), that might be discussed. The abuser needs to hear the pain and ongoing effect of those actions, taking responsibility for them. The abused sibling should remember, however, that the abuser also has a story to tell. What led that child to do such a thing?

On the other hand, pursuing contact with a sibling who is currently abusive, either verbally, emotionally, or physically, may be harmful. You may need to carefully assess when being in contact with your sibling is destructive. If that relationship can't be changed with professional help, then you need to come to peace with that reality—for now. Who knows what will happen between you two, however, in the next 20 to 30 years?

Men

"Since I had a sexual life for many years and happily explored that part of life, menopause felt like another stage. Not better or worse, just different." Gloria Steinem is talking here about a physical side of aging. "With myself, since menopause, that part of my brain that had always been a reliable home for sex is gone. It's gone! . . . I would have [thought] it's a loss. But it isn't. It's fine" (pp. 52–53).

Some women reach menopause and feel a release from the pressure of having to have a man, but many don't. Certainly, menopause may help you come to peace with your sexual drive, but it doesn't necessarily ease the intensity of wanting a partner. It doesn't address the old messages that might still be tucked away inside saying you must "find a man." It also is totally unrelated to skin hunger, your body's need for touch.

In preparation for old age, you have to come to some peace about men. This doesn't mean you have to give up hope of ever finding a man. There are always lovely reports of couples meeting and marrying in a retirement community or a nursing home.

No, giving up hope is not necessarily the same as coming to peace. You do have to find a way to live with the ambiguity, however, so you don't keep acting like the 20-year-old single you once were.

In preparation for old age, you need to acknowledge what you have learned about single men and about relating to them. Experience does count! Women who have been single for many years are quicker to recognize a "line" from a man than those inexperienced in the single world. They can rely on their prior history with other men.

After years of singles groups, dances, trips, and personal ads, you may have had enough. You may have moved men to the background, putting your energy into areas that are more rewarding and that give you a personal sense of satisfaction. Or you may have found a way to participate in the single experience, keeping it enjoyable and fresh, considering these events as part of your social activities. If you meet someone, fine. If not, at least you are enjoying yourself.

On the other hand, you may continue doing these things because that is what you feel you *must* do to prove you are trying to find a man. You return from singles events depressed, less self-confident, or having less respect for yourself. If this is true for you, continuing these activities may be self-abusive.

I once saw an Always Single woman in her late 60s flipping through the newspaper, looking for singles events for that weekend. I wondered how she felt doing what she had done for so many weekends over so many decades. Maybe she had difficulty seeing herself age because she didn't have the markers of seeing her children grow up. Maybe she just ignored noticing how she was moving to a new life stage. Whatever the reason, she continued looking for men in the same way she had been looking since she was a young woman.

For newly Single Agains, your most recent experience in the single world may have been when you were a teenager or young adult. You need practice in learning how to be a midlife single. You don't want to fall back on what you used to know about dating and men. That would keep you locked in a young adult position despite your maturity.

As a newly Single Again, your attending a singles dance, even if you have a bad time, can be an important learning experience as an adult. As one woman in my study said: "I've had some rotten dates, but I always come back afterward and ask myself: What can I learn from that? What could I do differently next time?"

You may need to have many experiences—at dances, through ads, with singles groups, etc.—in order to learn to maneuver around in the single world while maintaining your self-esteem.

There are no quick fixes for coming to peace with the ambiguity of not knowing if you will ever find a man. Each woman must find her own path for thinking about men as she gets older. One guideline may be useful, however: *respect yourself*. You may or may not be lucky enough to find a man, but you must always live with yourself.

Thinking about how you have changed already in relation to men may give you more insight into how you want to think about men as you age. Did you used to wait to make plans for the weekend, hoping a man would call? Did you change plans with a friend if you had an opportunity to be with a man? Were you as much yourself with him as you were with your female friends?

In your eagerness, did you too often "give him a chance" and "give him the benefit of the doubt"? Did you do this at the expense of ignoring the clues that he was not an appropriate man for you? Did you reinterpret the information you learned through being with him that didn't fit with what you wanted him to be?

As you age, you want to become better at reading men. You need to check your fantasies about them with the reality of what they are telling and showing you about themselves.

Reflection: How You Have Changed In Relation To Men

Think about the men you used to go out with when you were younger. Can you remember ways you waited for them, behaved with them, that you would not do today? Presumably, you have changed in many ways.

Make a list, and then admire how you have grown.

Now, think how you would handle each situation if it occurred today. Practice in your head the statements that you would make and how you would prefer to behave.

Preparing For Retirement

What's your fantasy about retirement? Luxuriating on the beach in a southern isle? Putzing around your house? Reading? Gardening? Playing with your grandchildren? No stockings, no high heels, no faxes, no e-mails? Starting a new business?

The original meaning of retirement was to retire *from* a job. It used to be we didn't have to explain how we spent our time. Over the past few decades, though, the trend is to retire *to* something. As soon as someone retires, the question is, "What are you going to *do?*

There's no one right way to think about retirement. For some women, retiring gives them the freedom to stop pushing so hard. They can pursue other areas of interest without having to worry about making a living. For other women, retirement seems impossible. "I'll never be able to afford it." They can't imagine having enough money to live without having to work, or they can't imagine being without the hustle and bustle of the work world.

You need to consider two issues as you prepare for retirement. First, your finances. Do you have enough money to stop working, or must you bring in money to support yourself? (See the section on financial preparation, below.) The other issue is thinking about the quality of life and the lifestyle you will want. Do you want to slow the pace of your life, or, conversely, invest more energy into whatever you plan next? Do you want to expand on what you've been doing, or do you want to put something different in your life?

Some women just want to retire, no questions asked. They consider this *their* time after years of doing their duty. It's their time to do all the things they've put off because they didn't have the time to focus on themselves: take a course in Yiddish, play golf, take acting classes, learn to knit, twiddle their thumbs.

Some women have their retirement planned before leaving their job. If you are in a job with a mandatory retirement age, your retirement package may be used as a startup for a new career.

Other women take a few years to settle in and see what comes next. The wonderful thing about retirement is, it's your choice!

Retirement is for when you are old, but if you don't know when old age starts, how do you know when you should retire? This is especially true for self-employed women who have no built-in age at which to stop working.

Whatever your thoughts about retirement, consider doing something that will feel meaningful to you. Ask yourself what you want to recall about your first decade of retirement, your second, your third. Personally, I don't know what I want yet, but I do know I want the rhythm of my life to be slower. I listen to Sharon's answering machine—"I'm sorry I'm not here. I'm out watching the water"—and I am envious.

Logistics Of Preparing For Old Age

Financial Preparation

Most of us women were raised to expect a husband to financially take care of us. Now, as we move toward old age, we find we're paying the price for this gender discrimination. During our 20s and 30s, when our brothers were saving and investing, we were spending our 60 cents to every one of their dollars on clothing, makeup, trips, books, and charitable contributions.

"I love what I do; I don't care whether I make a lot of money or not." This was the chant of women in my generation as we moved from college to low-paying jobs in teaching, nursing, social work. It never occurred to us, as it did to so many men, that it was okay to love what we did *and* get paid a lot of money to do it.

"In the United States, there's an epidemic of financial illiteracy, especially among women," says Doug Lewis, a certified financial planner *and* my older brother. It took him only 15 years to get me to listen to his sound advice about money.

The societal patriarchy that conveys "I'll take care of you" picks up after women move out of their parents' home. As Doug puts it, "They work in corporations that become surrogate fathers providing pensions; they have the government's Social Security. These are wonderful cushions, and many women need them for financial survival. But financial survival is not the same as financial independence. For this, you need to take care of yourself."

I'm lucky I listened to my brother before I had a crisis. Many women are not so lucky. They become aware of the importance of taking care of themselves as a result of a life crisis. That was the experience of Mary Donahue, coauthor of *On Your Own: A Widow's Passage to Emotional and Financial Well-Being* (Dearborn Financial Publishing, 1993). She was unexpectedly widowed at a young age. As a therapist, she had a good handle on dealing with the emotional components of her grief. But she was totally unprepared for the financial aspect of pulling her life together.

She hooked up with Alexandra Armstrong, a woman who was raised by a single mother. Armstrong understood early on the importance and power of money and became a successful certified financial planner so she could help others. Together, these women have written a guidebook that is useful not only for widows, but for any woman wanting to understand the basics of taking care of herself financially.

In their book, they say women need a financial planner, and they need to choose that person carefully, making sure they have the required credentials. Interview several; don't just go with the first one. Request an initial consultation (which often is free), and then ask lots of questions. For example:

- What is the hourly rate?

- Will I get a written estimate of the anticipated costs?

- If I select you, will you give me an itemized bill? How often will it be sent?

- Who takes the primary responsibility for the work, the professional or her assistant?

Make sure the professional knows you may occasionally have questions and you expect a return call—within at least one to two days. Make it clear you want the work done without unnecessary delays.

One of Armstrong and Donahue's practical suggestions is to consider hiring someone younger than you so that person can be your adviser for your lifetime. Now that's being prepared!

Yvette is teary eyed. "I know it's an irrational fear, but I'm scared of becoming a bag lady. I grew up in a family where money was very tight; both of my parents grew up in the Depression. You would think, then, that I'd have learned about investing and saving, but I haven't. Instead, I just live with this fear."

Neither Yvette, nor you, can change the past, but you can start making changes now. At the very least, arrange for a consultation with a financial planner who works on a fee basis, charging by the hour. Find out if financial independence is feasible for you, and, if not, what options you have to make it more possible.

When Yvette hears this advice, she says, "I can't afford that." Maybe not, but she never even called to price a consultation. Even if there is a fee, if you don't think you are worth the cost of that consultation, you may be committing financial suicide.

Many women think they can't understand financial matters. That's why you need a good professional who can explain it in simple terms. Doug explains investments in terms like chickens and eggs. If you are hungry and own a chicken, eat only the eggs because they keep coming. Never eat your chicken because it is what produces your eggs. Relating that image to money, don't touch your principal (the chicken) because that's what keeps producing the interest (the eggs).

Personally, I like these visuals. Yvette doesn't. "I need the hard facts, *if* I'm going to do this." She eventually did consult with a certified financial planner. Afterward, she reported: "Let's see if I have this correct. Step one: I need to know how much money it takes for me to live comfortably today. Step two: I need to translate what this amount will be in 15 years from now, the year I would like to stop working. That has to do with cost of living, or inflation.

"Step three: This amount will tell me how much money I need to be bringing in from my investments—not the total of the investments I have accumulated, but the income or growth that my investment makes. When the financial planner told me that amount, I thought I'd keel over! Apparently, though, it's still doable.

"Step four: That amount gets divided by the number of years from now until then. If every month from now till I'm 65 I send $200 to an individual retirement account—an IRA—she told me about, I'll be fine."

Yvette took a deep breath; she looked proud of herself for having recounted this. It seemed she really did understand.

She then continued. "I was all ready to say I couldn't possibly find $200 each month to stash away; I hardly ever have enough at the end of each month as it is. She said if I couldn't afford the $200 some month, I could send less or nothing at all. Nothing is written in stone.

"She gave me a cute little book called *The Wealthy Barber* [by David Chilton, Prima Publishing, 1997] and told me to read it. I had no intention of reading any of these wonderful books on financial stuff. I'm not interested. But as I flipped through the first few pages, I got caught up. It's like a novel, a story of a young couple going to visit the barbershop near their parents' summer vacation home. Before I knew it, I was really listening to the barber myself. I forget lots of the stuff, but the one thing that stayed with me was 'Pay yourself first.'"

Yvette got the one phrase that almost every book on finances emphasizes. Before you pay your utility bills, your credit card bill, or your department store bills, write a check to yourself. It's a variation on the scientific theory that you fill up whatever space you have; with money, you spend what you have. If you take your money for investments off the top, before you write any other check, you will still spend what you have, only you'll have saved some money first!

"Four weeks divided into $200. That's $50 a week," Yvette calculated. "If I write myself a check every week for $50, that seems so doable. I write lots of $50 checks each month, why not some for me?" Yvette was actually excited about this discovery. "All I have to do now is keep remembering the amount of money I will have with that $50 a week accumulating, and making more money for the next 15 years. That may be a big enough motivator to get me to keep doing this. That little $50 may be my ticket to being financially independent so I can retire when I want!"

For many women, $50 a week is not doable. However, saving even $1 a week will accumulate a lot more than not saving anything at all! And, when you reach 62 or 65, you'll be glad you saved whatever amount you did.

In their book, Armstrong and Donahue aptly quote Yogi Berra: "You've got to be careful if you don't know where you're going, because you might not get there"! In preparing for your old age, you do need to know if you can financially take care of yourself, so you'll be able to get there. This is another form of taking control of your life.

Legal Preparation

As a large percentage of our population ages, certain attorneys are specializing in gerontological law. Many bar associations have committees for members who practice "elder law." There is even a National Academy of Elder Law Attorneys.

As you prepare for aging, you should consider the following few standard issues to protect yourself and your estate—that's the legal term for your possessions, property, and savings—in case you become incapable of handling your own financial and health matters. They are: wills, living wills, health care power of attorney, general power of attorney, long-term care insurance, and property protection.

Wills

I'm indebted to my friend and colleague Barbara Beach, Esq., for much of the information in this section. In discussions with her, I've learned that a will can be complex or simple, depending on your possessions and property. Before her financial consultation, Yvette said, "I don't need a will yet." Many women say the same thing: "Wills are for old people." Actually, that's not quite accurate. Wills are for anyone who may someday die!

Whether or not to write a will depends on several considerations. Do you have strong feelings about who should inherit your money and possessions? Do you have strong feelings about being buried or cremated? Do you have a pet you want to provide for after your death? If your estate is large, do you have strong feelings about paying Uncle Sam taxes?

If you have answered "Yes" to any of these questions, you need a will. Making a will in advance can save you and your heirs time, hassles, and money. Your estate will be taxed after you die; much of its value will go to Uncle Sam if you aren't prepared. Also, it may be several years before your relatives receive the family heirlooms or that great watercolor over your sofa. Without a will, legal rigmarole can tie up your possessions for a long time, causing a financial and time imposition on your family.

To find an attorney, ask your friends who prepared their will. Was their attorney easy to work with, responding promptly to their phone calls? If you decide to secure a will, make sure it is drafted by an attorney licensed in your state, since some states have different laws. A will may be invalid if it is not written correctly, and, unfortunately, you will not be able to correct any mistakes.

The cost of a will can range anywhere from $100 to thousands of dollars, so be a smart customer. Most attorneys charge a flat rate for a will. Make sure you know beforehand what that rate covers.

Wills must have an executor, the person responsible for carrying out the deceased's requests. You can choose anyone you want, a relative or friend, an attorney, even a bank.

Living Will

If you are critically ill, under what conditions do you want to be kept alive? Do you want to be put on a life support system, or do you want to be allowed to die without heroic medical efforts? Whom do you trust to make that decision? You've heard the media stories about family members fighting with the doctors and the courts. It's a shame living wills aren't mandatory.

Many attorneys recommend against naming your physician as the decision maker because that medical professional should advise your representative, not make the decisions.

Health Care Power Of Attorney

This document states that you give your permission for someone else to legally represent your wishes about medical procedures (other than life support ones) in case you can't do it yourself. This becomes especially important if your relatives disagree about what, if any, treatment you should be given.

General Power Of Attorney

This document gives a person power to handle your financial affairs and pay your bills, and anything else that you have listed in the document. A power of attorney will continue in effect even if you become mentally incompetent if it contains language specifying your wish that it should be so. (This is a "durable" power of attorney.) A power of attorney terminates upon your death because your affairs will then be handled by your estate—whether or not you made a will.

Many attorneys advise you to keep the document designating the person who holds your general power of attorney, or you should leave it with your attorney, rather than give it to the person you've chosen. This way, if you change your mind about whom you want to have your power of attorney, you don't have to retrieve it. Also, this protects you from its being misused.

Long-Term Care Insurance

Years ago this was considered a luxury. Not so today. Until our government is clearer about how to help ill seniors, you need to prepare to take care of yourself. Many different types of long-term care insurance policies are available, so interview a number of agents. You want to be sure the company has a solid financial record because you want it to be in existence if you ever need it. It is cheaper to buy it while you are younger. Don't wait until you need long-term care insurance before looking into it!

Property Protection

Tax laws have become more people friendly in some areas, and this is one. If you want someone in particular to have your home after you die, you can add his or her name to the deed now. That may protect your property if you go to a nursing home that requires you to spend all your assets before they reduce the monthly costs.

Be aware of the drawbacks to this, however. One is that you can't sign for a new mortgage, sell the house, or get a home equity loan without that person's agreement.

Preparing For Your Death

If you have signed a will, you have legally prepared for your death. It is a good idea to make a list of what you want your executor (or if you have no will, your next of kin) to do when you die. Make sure you tell everyone where that list is, so they can find it if you die unexpectedly.

While you are in good health, you might also consider making funeral and burial arrangements, like picking out a burial plot, casket, headstone. This makes it easier on your next of kin, so they don't have to deal with those issues while they are coping with their grief over your death.

Standing over my aunt's grave a few years ago led me to wonder about single women and burials. When you have a husband, you are usually buried together. When you don't, then where will you be buried? In your childhood hometown, or in a town where you lived as an adult?

On the other hand, do single women avoid that decision by choosing cremation? Do they do so because they don't want to be buried alone, don't know which site to choose, don't think anyone would visit their gravesite? This is an issue no one has seriously explored, yet. However, more people today than ever before are opting for cremation, for a variety of reasons.

If cremation is your preference, have you considered if you want your ashes strewn somewhere special, or buried? If you want your body donated to science, have you made arrangements for that?

The women in my study showed slightly more interest in being cremated than in being buried or having their bodies donated to science. Those who wanted to be buried didn't seem to worry about other people's reactions to their spending eternity next to their parents.

Only one woman minded. "I don't want people to say, 'There lies an old spinster who even in death has to be with her parents.'" Most women, though, said things like: "That's where I belong." "I won't care; I'll be dead." "If I'm still single when I die, where else would I be buried?" "Mother has space for me." "Great! I'd be at home."

Do you avoid thinking about preparing for your death? One woman half-jokingly said: "One good reason to get married is so I don't have to worry about this. We'll have a family plot and that's that!"

Preparing for your old age is one other way to take charge of your life. You have no control over finding an emotionally available man, but as with all the other tasks, you can take control over how you chose to deal with your aging.

Self-Assessment

The eighth task, Preparing for Old Age, involves five key issues. Look them over to see how you are doing in each one.

Coming To Grips With An Identity As An Older Single Woman

Preparing Relationships With
___your children
___your friends
___your siblings

Coming To Peace Around The Issue Of Men

Preparing For Retirement

Preparing For The Logistics Of Aging
___finances
___wills
___living wills
___health care power of attorney
___general power of attorney
___long-term care insurance
___property protection
___burial

For any category that you are satisfied with, give yourself a "star," either figuratively or literally. For any that you still need to work on, think about what needs to be added or changed in order for it to be satisfactory. Then, write your ideas for that category.

If you are stuck, talk with friends or family to see how they handle that task. If you are still stuck after that, consider reading a self-help book, taking a course that deals with the topic, or talking with a professional: for example, a gerontologist; a professional counselor; a religious leader; an attorney who specializes in issues for the elderly; a financial planner; and a life insurance (long-term insurance) agent.

13

Teaching Men

Tara was married to Greg for 20 years. The 10 years since her divorce have given her plenty of time to reflect on both married and single life. Thinking back over the single men she has met, she wonders if she made a mistake in divorcing Greg. "Maybe that was as good as it gets."

Adjusting Your Expectations

Tara was born to lower-middle-class parents whose family had lived in Kansas for six or seven generations. The men and women married their high school sweethearts, bought homes in the same town, and raised their children expecting the same for them. As the next to the youngest of six children, she had no reason to expect anything different for herself.

Following family tradition, Tara married Greg, literally the boy next door. His mother was married to her father's first cousin. A month after the marriage, they rented a third-cousin's home and Greg worked for his father's second cousin by marriage. Tara had her first child a year and a half later. After the second child, she started using birth control, unbeknownst to Greg. (Tara swore the doctor, someone else's first or third cousin, to secrecy.) Greg was extremely successful in his cousin's business; soon the family moved to a big city on the other side of the state to open another store, which also prospered.

From the vantage point of who she is today, Tara thinks of Greg as a man who was "generous, sometimes to a fault." He made a lot of money and bought her gifts—jewelry, clothing, anything she asked for, or didn't even think to ask for. He belonged to all the right clubs, and they were socially very active. He had many friends, and everyone who knew him said he was kind.

In the 15 years they lived there, Tara could remember just one time when they went out to dinner together—alone. At first the excitement of this life was enough for her, a small town woman. But it soon wore thin. She was "his wife," an extension of his success. She was not supposed to work ("It wouldn't look good"). He took very good care of her. They didn't have many fights, and he was a reasonably good lover.

"So why did you leave?" I ask.

"I wanted more intimacy. I complained, and he didn't seem to understand or want to understand what I wanted. I wanted something more personal from him: not just talking about feelings, but talking about politics, literature, anything that was a real exchange between us. Greg was so superficial.

"Then there was that fatal trip. I arranged a special weekend. It was the most romantic event I could plan. It included the wining and dining he loved and time for us to cuddle up in bed, go for long walks, sit in the sun—all with lots of time for talking and sharing. I even brought a book I knew he'd enjoy, so we could read together. I was in seventh heaven.

"On Sunday night, when we got home, I was unpacking, preparing us for getting back to the real world. Greg came into the bedroom. He wasn't smiling, but he wasn't frowning, either, so I had no reason to think anything special about it.

"'I've done it now, Tara,'" he said. "'I gave you the weekend you wanted. I was as intimate as I know how. Now, don't ever ask for that again.'

"He wasn't mad. He might have been telling me he tried a new dish I prepared and didn't really like it. I was so surprised, I just nodded. But that night, after he fell asleep, I lay there for hours crying. I was hurt, but more, I was scared. I knew I had to do something. The next morning I started planning the divorce."

Tara expected that if Greg just had the opportunity to be intimate, if she could just show him how, he would *want* it. She personalized Greg's response, assumed it was her job to make that happen.

Greg obviously loved Tara very much. When she planned this trip, he knew what she wanted, and he tried it. He sat on the beach, at dinner, in bed and talked with her. They read together. He discussed how much they loved each other, dreamed about their future together. They cuddled and made love. He did not play golf or leave her by herself at any point.

For him, the trip was stressful and tiring. There was nothing really enjoyable about it other than knowing he was pleasing Tara. "I'm not that kind of guy. I don't like talking much. I like to keep busy." He certainly didn't feel any closer to her; in fact, "I felt strained the whole time."

Many women need emotional intimacy and a more personal connection with a man. Some, like Tara, expect a man to have the same need. If he doesn't, they personalize his lack of interest, assuming they have somehow failed. They may ponder what actually is an irrelevant question: Is it he *won't* or *can't* be more intimate? If you open a new door for a man, give him lots of encouragement and guidance on how to enter it, and are willing to renegotiate how far the door should open, yet the man still isn't interested in going through the door, there's nothing you can do. It's irrelevant if he won't or can't.

For some women, emotional intimacy from a man is at the top of their need list. They can't make major adjustments in their expectations; to do so would be to deny themselves something *significantly important,* to risk damaging their self-esteem.

Some women would like intimacy, but they need other qualities from a partner more. Ronnie knew before she married a second time that her husband, Burt, would never be comfortable with sharing his feelings or responding to hers. They would never have personal discussions about anything—themselves, other people, real-life events. But he provided companionship and a financial security that were of far greater importance to her.

They've had a comfortable five years together. Sometimes she feels lonely and regrets how emotionally disconnected they are. She rarely talks to him about anything personal. Yet, she always comes back to thinking about the satisfying life they have together. Did she make a mistake in giving up intimacy to be with Burt? She replies: "No. Life is full of compromises. You can't get all you want, and companionship is more important to me. I can always talk with my girlfriends."

The absence of emotional intimacy doesn't have to be fatal to a relationship. As Ronnie decided, it just means that a woman has to readjust what she expects from a partner. She is settling, but without the negative connotation of compromising herself. Since you know you can't get everything you want in a man, settling just means taking charge of the areas in which you are willing to compromise yourself. If your personality style does not *demand* emotional intimacy from a man, consider yourself lucky. By removing your expectation that a man participate in personal discussions, a wider range of men will be available to you.

However, for women whose personality does require emotional intimacy, there may be little room for compromise. You may have fewer options among men. Thinking about it this way, Tara realizes that without a certain degree of emotional intimacy with a man, she feels depressed. She didn't realize that while she was married to Greg. If she had stayed in that marriage, she would have de-pressed an important need and been really miserable. That marriage may have been as good as it gets, and for some women, it would have been enough. But she decides she needs more intimacy or—and this is difficult for her to own—she can't be with a man.

"I must stay honest with myself. I've dated enough men now to know I won't be happy with a man who can't relate to me this way. There has to be someone like that out there, and if not, I'd rather be without a man and content with my life than with a man and miserable."

For women thinking about leaving a marriage or relationship, I often use the crystal ball exercise. If you could look into a crystal ball and see that you would never meet a man with more emotional availability than the one you currently are with, what would you do? Would you rather stay with him anyway, or would you still choose to leave him?

On days when Ronnie is annoyed at Burt, she envisions her crystal ball and feels assured. Tara also uses this exercise to reassure herself. She's disappointed she hasn't met a more appropriate man, apprehensive if she ever will. Even so, she's glad she left Greg and is willing to take her chances on meeting someone else. Staying with him was suffocating an essential part of her.

If you are like Ronnie, you can be content with adjusting your expectations in a man and settling for one who offers you more of the qualities you require—even if not intimacy. If you are like Tara, you may not be willing to compromise your need for intimacy, so you keep looking and remain satisfied with your life in the process.

Basically, you do not have many choices about this; either you need emotional intimacy in order to be with a man, or you accept a man with other characteristics and find intimacy elsewhere. One way is no better or worse than the other. Which of these choices works best for you is related to your personality; hence, there may be little you can do to change this. If being single did not carry with it such a negative connotation, women would not feel the pressure to squeeze themselves into a relationship that didn't meet their essential needs.

Pseudo-Intimacy

Most people have expectations about what they want in a relationship, and then choose a partner to fulfill those expectations. During the early infatuation of a romance, both women and men fall in love with their fantasy of who the other person is. This is called pseudo-intimacy. It looks and feels like genuine intimacy, but it can't be because genuine intimacy takes time.

Arguments and dissatisfaction often occur as a result of one or both partners feeling betrayed in discovering their illusions about the other person. Real intimacy can come only after you've successfully handled anger with each other and resolved the fights. You both learn you can be forthright and say what you need to say; you can fight cleanly; and you can resolve the fight in a way that leaves you both feeling good about yourselves and about your relationship. Real intimacy can come only if, after the illusions have been broken, you still want the person—warts and all. Many couples never get to this level of genuine intimacy.

Shoebox Vs. The Mantel

Another area where expectations must be adjusted relates to what men and women do with their caring feelings. During the "courting" period, a man may very much be the romantic pursuer. But, as the newly single Tara discovered, and you may have experienced: "That stops as soon as a man knows you're interested. It's as if he's only interested in the hunt, not the catch."

You think he's no longer as interested in you because he doesn't continue behaving the way he had. He no longer expresses his feelings; he doesn't call as often as he used to; he doesn't bring you little things like he did during the infatuation period. "It's almost as if he takes me for granted," explains Tara.

That may not be the case. There may be a simple explanation for his change that has little to do with his not being interested in you. It has to do with shoeboxes. When a man owns something special, something he values greatly, he wraps it carefully, lovingly, and tucks it in a shoebox, which he then slides under his bed. He leaves it there, knowing it is safe and close at hand. He can think about it as much as he likes—at home or work or anytime—because he knows where it is. He doesn't have to go there and open it up to look at it.

Contrast this with a woman who owns something special. She showcases it on the mantel. She goes there frequently to dust it, rearrange it, just to look at and admire it, and she wants others to see it and admire it.

Because these two styles are so different, they may breed disappointment. It's often not enough for a woman to know the man thinks about her but doesn't bother letting her know. She can try teaching him what she needs to hear (see Chapter 9), but she should at least acknowledge, not discount, his style, which has value for *him*.

Turnoffs

You should set limits, though, as to how much you can adjust your expectations about a man. You certainly don't want to adjust them to accept physical, sexual, verbal, or emotional abuse, nor disrespect of you as a person or as a woman. There are murky areas, however, such as turnoff behaviors that are not abusive but nonetheless unappealing to women.

"Some men just don't get it. Don't they understand how they turn us off?" asks Emily. I hear many variations of this question. The answer probably is *no*. As long as a woman protects a man's ego, not saying why she is not interested in him, he may have no way of knowing that his self-centered conversation, or crude comments, or condescension is a turnoff. From my preliminary study of single men (see Chapter 9), it seems that many men really may not have a good understanding of how they turn off women, why they can't find a partner.

When Ryan returns to his apartment after an evening with Emily, he shrugs, feeling confused. He just met this woman for a drink. He thinks they had a good time. He certainly enjoyed her. She's sexy, has a great figure. She laughs a lot and seems really smart. "So why," he questions, "did she refuse to see me again?"

If Emily had heard Ryan's question, she would have been appalled. She would have wondered if he were deaf. How much clearer could she possibly have been? According to her version: "We got together for coffee after work, and after an hour and a half, I *needed* to go home. It was so awful. When he asked if he could see me the next night, I took a deep breath and said: 'No. I don't want to see you again. Frankly, I didn't enjoy myself tonight. You either talked about yourself, or you were silent. You asked nothing about me, and showed no interest in me until you wanted to kiss me. Why would I want to give up another night to be with you? You mentioned you hoped to get married again some day. So, if you do this with other women, consider this a friendly piece of information.'

"Was I polite? I don't know. But *I* felt better afterward."

Even with her friendly piece of information, Ryan doesn't understand that his behavior had turned Emily off. As a therapist, I see too many men who are just as obtuse as Ryan. Emily's comment would not motivate them toward self-reflection. Some might go home feeling unfairly attacked by her; some might have a beer and call it a bad evening. Presumably, though, some men would give serious consideration to what Emily said, wondering what they could do that would be more effective in relating to women.

Should a woman speak up when a man does something that is a big turnoff? Many women say, "Why bother?" But I suggest you think about it as altruism for men and for other women. If enough women bothered, you might meet some of the recipients who took those women's candor seriously.

Kim was immediately attracted to Art when they met at a gallery benefit. They arranged to have dinner the following week. During dinner, though, Art talked about himself nonstop. He was interesting, but Kim was annoyed. "I went to the ladies room, to give me time to think. I decided I had two choices. If I decided not to say anything, for sure I wouldn't want to see him again. My other choice was to tell him what he was doing. The only reason for doing that, I reasoned, was if he could hear how self-absorbed he was and begin to show more interest in talking with me (not at me), then he might be a man worth my getting to know.

"I went back to the table and decided, 'What the hell.' I told him my two choices. He was really surprised and appreciative. He said, 'No one has cared enough to tell me I run on at the mouth. Thanks.' That was the start of a very nice (but not perfect) relationship. We had a good year together, and our decision to break up was a result of our good communication."

Kim benefited by her speaking up. And so did Art. (And so, hopefully, did the next woman in Art's life.) If women don't speak up, men may never learn.

Another type of turnoff is a man's one-upmanship. While it fits his socialization among males, as we saw in Chapter 9, it doesn't work well with women. When a man accepts that "when someone criticizes or complains about you, you criticize or complain about them harder; and the one who retaliates the hardest wins," he probably has no idea what an awful turnoff that is. Yet, if your only choices are to be the one on the top or the one on the bottom, it makes sense you'll go for the top.

When we consider the gender-specific messages men have received over their lifetime, turnoff behaviors make sense. If a man is not a winner, he is a loser. What man would willingly opt for being a loser? Terrance Real's explanation about grandiosity (see Chapter 9) is useful in understanding men's turnoff behaviors with women. Men vacillate between shame and grandiosity. A woman's request for sharing stirs the very feelings a man defends against, that cause shame. Men present their toughened side to the world, especially to women. In some men, this toughened side may be exhibited through grandiosity—sounding pompous, lecturing to, not talking with, women. When you bump into men's turnoff behaviors, you probably are bumping into their efforts to ward off their emotional side, protecting their vulnerability.

Teaching Tools

The ability to make a relationship work, like any other job, requires specific skills and techniques. Yet, unlike becoming a scientist, a beautician, or a salesperson, you have no school or specialized training to choose from for the important job of having a healthy loving relationship.

What training men and women do get comes mostly from childhood, watching how your parents treated each other. It's the lucky child who sees mutual respect and good communication. But a boy may see his mother cater to the father, cower from him, discount her needs in favor of his; he may see his father bully or withdraw from his mother. This boy may vow, as a child, that he'll be entirely different when he grows up. Even while saying that, he's unconsciously absorbing what's expected of him as a man.

Despite detesting that behavior, when he reaches adulthood, he finds his parents' type of relationship familiar. If he hasn't dealt with the loyalty issues with his parents, he may find himself repeating the very things he swore he'd never do.

The same situation is true for women. They may find themselves repeating a familiar type of relationship even though they said they'd be different. (Remember Beth in Chapter 11?) One major difference between men and women, though, is that many women spend time thinking, reading, and talking to friends about relationships and self-improvement. Women are more likely than men to seek therapy to resolve issues from their childhood. Hence, by midlife, women have probably had some training in making a relationship work.

It is not surprising, then, that it is the woman (usually, but not always) who becomes the communication teacher in a relationship. A generalization that has some merit is that men believe if a situation isn't broken, tinkering with it could make it worse. They would tinker only if there was an imminent threat of losing a woman. Women, though, perceive a partnership without communicating as a problem, and they tinker to make it better. Therefore, they are more likely to say, "We need to talk."

In all good relationships, partners do teach each other. Each offers different arenas of expertise. Men usually are the career mentors, teaching and encouraging a woman to reach higher professionally. Women usually are the relationship mentors, teaching a man to recognize when a problem exists and how to fix it. When teaching is accepted by both people as valuable, you both benefit. The men who are willing to engage in the learning process are generally those who are already involved with a woman and don't want to lose her. A man who is just getting to know a woman doesn't have the bond to hold him, so he may walk away from self-reflection and working out the problems.

As I use the term here, *teaching* includes expressing your needs clearly and directly, and then suggesting different ways a man can respond to you. In Chapter 9 we looked at guidelines for expressing your needs. In this section, we'll consider four tools for teaching men how to talk with you. These are: engaging in emotional foreplay, switching shoes, playing verbal tennis, and red-flagging intimidation.

Engaging In Emotional Foreplay

Emotional foreplay is a woman's aphrodisiac: it is sexually exciting and increases desire. It's a turn-on. Many men, however, mistakenly think the primary aphrodisiac for women is sex, nurtured along with romance. They may be surprised, therefore, when their best efforts to be romantic don't win a woman's heart. They don't understand that this is *not* what turns a woman on.

By midlife, women know that candlelight dinners, romantic trips, and even the proverbial diamonds are lovely, but they can fade as fast as the candles burn down. They may add to a glowing heart, but the wick must first be lit. And that wick, for many women, is communication and personal sharing.

"Fred never got it," says Fran about the man she calls her "most recent ex-almost-beau. It's real easy to turn me on. I need a four-letter word, but not the same four letters he was talking about. Maybe he was overly impressed that both our names are a four-letter F word. But the four-letter word that turns me on doesn't start with an F. It starts with a T, for t-a-l-k."

The best aphrodisiac for many, but not all, women is something that helps a woman feel emotionally connected with a man. It can be talking about feelings or sharing personal experiences. "It's certainly not how much money a man makes, hearing him talk about himself, or prattling on about his friends," exclaims Fran.

There's an old anonymous saying that men feel intimate as a result of making love, whereas women need to feel intimate *before* they want to make love. This captures yet another of the many communication problems between men and women, which is why both sexes need to be bilingual, knowing what motivates and pleases their partner as well as themselves.

Fran, long since over Fred, puzzles: "How come men don't understand that women need emotional foreplay before that other stuff? It works on me every time!"

Switching Shoes

When I was a child, I used to see a sign posted around town: "A family that prays together stays together." If we adapt that to relationships, it would say, "A couple that fights together stays together. . . as long as they fight productively."

One of the biggest problems in getting to know a man (as well as in sustaining an ongoing relationship) is dealing with conflict. Many people try to avoid confronting it, saying, "I don't want to start a fight; I don't want to upset him/her." Yet, the very act of avoiding the tension usually leads to more tension and bigger problems. Most arguments can't and shouldn't be avoided. Speaking up when you have uncomfortable feelings actually *decreases* the fighting—as long as it is done in a clean manner.

Some arguments result from misunderstandings and others from a genuine difference of opinion. But they never have to be *an attack on the person.* If you can keep to the issue, if you are confident that you both *want* to resolve the issue, if you feel respect for the other person, then *arguments can actually enhance a relationship,* bringing two people closer.

In most discussions, the issue doesn't have to be who's right or wrong. It's easy to assume that both parties believe they are right: people don't usually push their point knowing they are wrong! Getting *inside the other's shoes* helps you both understand how the other came to that point of view.

A few weeks after I start seeing Jerry, I am telling him something interesting that I learned in my recent trip to Russia. I had been standing on one of the St. Petersburg bridges, talking with an artist who was putting the finishing touches on his painting of the Church of the Bleeding Resurrection. I had asked if he were Russian. He had replied, "Yes, but my mother was Jewish."

I am telling Jerry I had wondered why the artist made that distinction, and I am getting ready to explain what I later learned: even if you were born in Russia, if your parents or grandparents were Jewish, you still were identified as Jewish, not Russian.

But before I can say any of this, Jerry says, "I'll tell you why," and he starts to explain. I interrupt, saying, "I'll be glad to hear that, but first I want to finish my story." He gets huffy; for the life of me (remember, this is my version), I can't figure out why. We are now in an argument.

Repeatedly I tell him I didn't ask him a question; he repeatedly insists I cut him off. We aren't getting anywhere, except angrier at each other. I finally suggest trying to get inside each other's shoes to see if we can get past this. He agrees. I go first.

"You thought I asked you a question, then I didn't want to hear what were saying. Do I have that right?"

"Yep."

"From inside your shoes, I can see why you would be annoyed. Now see if you can get inside my shoes."

"You were telling me a story and I interrupted you. You didn't know I thought you asked me a question."

It was only when we both could be in the other's shoes that we realized we were having two unrelated conversations. Once we did, it was easy to see how we ended up in an argument and how to get out of it.

This was our first argument. As we were switching shoes and sorting out the who-said-what's, I felt a real warmth for Jerry. Apparently, he felt the same for me. Weeks later, when we'd become closer, I asked what he thought helped us get unstuck that evening.

After reflecting on his answer, Jerry explained: "Having us stand in each other's shoes was a real stretch. I didn't know if that made sense, but you made it clear that we didn't have to figure out who was right or wrong. That helped me get around the hurdle of my defensiveness."

Standing in each other's shoes removed the need for a winner and a loser. Without that one-upmanship tension, Jerry could focus on the issue we were discussing.

As he puts it: "I said to myself, 'She's worth getting to know better, so I'm willing to stretch.' If I hadn't thought you were worth getting to know better, I don't know that I would have bothered. You offered me a different way of solving the fight."

What typically happens in these types of arguments is that both people try harder to be heard. The more they feel unheard, the more they push their point of view. Then, no one hears much of anything!

When a couple comes into my office, I always face each one individually and affirm, "I will listen to your version of the problem, or situation, and I will believe you are 100 percent correct." Then, to the two of them as a couple, I add, "The fact that your two versions don't sound like you were in the same room, to say nothing of even being on the same planet, is why you are here." That sets the stage for removing rights and wrongs and prepares them for hearing what is in the other one's head.

When Carrie (whom we met in Chapter 9) said to Allen, after they returned from a lovely walk, "We have to talk," Allen felt attacked and snapped, "Why do you have to ruin everything?" How she responded to him would affect the direction of what came next in their conversation. She could have snapped back, or she could have said: "Let me try to understand what you think I just said. Your reaction suggests you may have not understood what I intended. Can you tell me what you heard me say?"

This would allow Allen to say, "You said we had this wonderful time together, and then you challenged me with your 'We have to talk.'" If he were switching shoes, he would have asked, "Is that right?"

Given that chance, Carrie could then respond: "Not quite. I said we had this wonderful time together and that I was feeling so close to you that I wanted to talk about our living together." They may have ended this conversation with a big chuckle and a hug instead of feeling attacked.

A basic requirement for standing in each other's shoes is to trust that the other person isn't out to "get" you. If you take that as your starting point, then it is easier to *want* to figure out what the other person could possibly have had in mind. Switching shoes works in communication between any two (or more) people, regardless of sex and the type of relationship.

Playing Verbal Tennis

We're sitting in the Acropolis, a neighborhood Greek restaurant. Melissa and I are relatively new friends, so there's much I don't know about her.

She's telling me an abbreviated version about herself and her partner, Eric. They've been together now for two years and are planning to marry—sometime, no hurry. "It's really an easy relationship now. We have so many common interests, and what's really special is how well we communicate—most of the time. But it wasn't always this way. I had to teach him to play tennis."

"What?" I exclaim. It's a reasonable question, given her apparent change of topics.

"He didn't know how to have a conversation with me. It was always one-sided. Either he'd talk and leave no space for me, or I'd be telling him something, and he'd just sit there saying nothing, as if not interested. I worried about this. Then I realized he just didn't know that conversations should go back and forth—like a tennis match. I hit the ball to him, and I expect him to hit it back to me. Then, I'll return it to him. Sometimes we hit the ball directly back to each other, like being on the same topic, and sometimes we hit it across court, like changing the topic. But we're in the game together. Now," Melissa continues, "if he starts a one-sided monologue, or if he doesn't respond when I'm talking, I just say 'Tennis.'"

This may sound elementary, but some men really don't realize a conversation has a rhythm. Melissa's analogy is a creative way to help them understand how women converse. It's visual and concrete.

Not knowing the rhythm is one explanation for why men don't play verbal tennis. Another explanation is that it doesn't occur to many men to ask a question. In their head, they believe: "If she wants to tell me something, she will. I shouldn't have to ask."

Knowing why a man doesn't participate more equitably in a conversation helps you choose the right approach for teaching him. Melissa knew Eric didn't have the rhythm, so she taught him.

Carrie knew Allen never thought about asking more about her, or when he did, he felt dumb or inadequate trying to figure out what to say. Therefore, she started giving him the words she wanted to hear—in everyday conversations as well as the more serious ones. For instance, after having told him about a meeting she attended, she would say, "I'd really like it if you'd ask me, 'What was it about?' or 'How did it go?' Sure, I could just tell you, but when you ask me questions about what I'm doing, it makes me feel you are interested in me and my world."

As Carrie and Allen end their therapy, she reflects on one of the things that helped improve their relationship. "When I'd be upset about something, Allen would get real quiet. I'd want to talk, but he withdrew. He said he didn't know what to say to make me feel better. Well, I *did* know what he could say, so I'd tell him. We aren't talking heavy-duty stuff here. I wanted something as simple as, 'What do you need right now?'

"At first he felt I was controlling by telling him what to say, and I couldn't understand why he wouldn't just say it to me. So what if I gave him the words; he didn't know what to say, and these were the words I wanted to hear. So, for goodness' sake, try it! He has, and it really makes a difference now."

A third explanation for why men drop the tennis ball of conversation is that they may be emotionally flooded. This can be a problem even for a long-time married man who is deeply committed to his wife.

Sarah and Saul have been married for almost 60 years. Sarah became progressively angry at Saul after her mastectomy. "Saul obviously doesn't care about what I've been through because he never mentions it to me." She insisted they go for therapy because she was worried her growing anger might lead her to the divorce court, "and I didn't want that after all these years."

In the session Sarah turns to him, first pleading and, when she gets no response, then fuming: "I want you to ask me about it. Anything!"

Saul sits silently, looking terribly uncomfortable. When I ask about his silence, Saul looks at her with eyes full of tears. "Of course I care. I was worried to death for you. I don't know what to say. I can't make it better." Men fix problems, and since this was one Saul couldn't fix, he felt shamed at being so helpless; then he became emotionally stifled.

I have Sarah dictate what she would like him to say to her. She comes up with four sentences for Saul to write down:

Are you scared the cancer will come back?

Are you in pain?

Would you like to talk about it?

I love you anyway, even with only one breast.

Saul tucked the paper in his shirt pocket, and during the next week, three times a day he pulled it out and asked her one of the questions.

You might consider this exercise to be artificial and corny, but it did provide a way for Saul to get used to the idea of talking to Sarah about the mastectomy. Soon, he no longer needed her questions; he was asking his own, including the one that worried him the most, "Can we still make love?"

Red-Flagging Intimidation

Intimidation has no one definition. What intimidates one woman has no affect on another. However, when you are feeling intimidated, you need to speak up. Too often, a man is totally surprised to find out what a powerfully negative effect he is having on a woman. Two of the more typical forms of intimidation are a man's voice and his facial expressions.

James is shocked when Jill, a woman he's been seeing for a few months, reveals, "You scare me when you get angry; I'm afraid you'll lose control and hurt me."

"What the hell are you talking about?" he screams (or so Jill thinks). "First off, I'm not angry, and second, even if I were, I'd never hurt you."

Jill cringes more, and in a timid voice, says, "You see what I mean?"

James's reaction is probably similar to many men's, just as many women will identify with Jill's reaction. I have James and Jill stand up next to one another and ask their height and weight. They laugh. James is 6'3" tall and weighs 250 pounds; Jill is 5'7" and weighs 153 pounds. While still standing, they record their voices, and then we play the tape back. Not surprising, James's voice is loud and deep; Jill's is soft and sounds almost thin. Last, I give James a mirror and have him make a face, as if he's mad.

When they sit down, James muses, "I see a pattern here." Jill doesn't have the words to explain what James is viscerally able to comprehend: his body size, deep voice, and intense facial expression make him appear scary to Jill. She is especially sensitive to this since she grew up with a physically and verbally abusive father.

Most men would be surprised at how often their voice and facial expressions scare a woman, particularly during an intense discussion, or if he swears or uses belittling language. Therefore, unless you have information to the contrary, err on the side of assuming that a man doesn't mean to frighten you. At a quiet time, when he is attentive, let him know that the volume of his voice and the expression on his face frighten you. He may say he isn't screaming. Don't argue the point; it's irrelevant. He just needs to hear *how it makes you feel.*

Then talk with him about what you can do when you are feeling intimidated by his voice. Some men like a hand signal; others prefer a statement like, "Would you mind lowering your voice?" Some couples have fun using a code word, such as "turnip greens" (or some other least favorite vegetable). The humor of that word popping up in the middle of an argument breaks the tension while reminding him to lower his voice.

If, in a new relationship, the man is not responsive after you have explained your feelings, then you may be learning something important about him. Ask yourself whether you are getting *from* him what you need. Is he worthy of you?

After using these four teaching tools, and keeping in mind the tips for talking with men that were explained in Chapter 9, you may find a man is quite pleased with the new way he expresses himself. Those men who are annoyed and unwilling to learn probably are not men who deserve you.

When To Retire From Teaching

A woman runs the risk of trying too hard and working overtime without reaping the benefits as she teaches a man how to communicate better. Or, conversely, she might be so successful that the man is uncomfortable staying with his "teacher," and he moves on to use his new skills with someone else.

Sonya and Hannah are having lunch in one of their favorite coffee shops. They are catching up on each other's lives since they haven't seen each other in a few months. Sonya is telling her friend how Nick "dumped" her.

"We had been together about five months. He was wonderful, loving, and generous. More important, he was willing, even eager, to learn how to talk and share his feelings with me. Then, last week, for no apparent reason, he tearfully tells me he loves me so much, but it wasn't 'that kind of love'! Then he left. I don't get it. This is the third man who has done this to me. You know what's going to happen now? I bet Nick marries the next woman he gets involved with. That's what the other two men did."

Hannah nods. "I know just what you mean. What is it with men? Ben, remember him? Well, he told me how much I helped him learn about himself, that he knows I'm responsible for his having grown so much. He said he'd be eternally devoted to me. Then he told me he needed to break up. He even had the audacity to ask if we could remain good friends. Who is he kidding!"

Two women sitting at a neighboring table must have been listening because they smiled, moving their heads up and down in exaggerated motion, as if confirming, "We know *exactly* what you mean!"

Sonya laughs by way of acknowledging them and goes on. "It really burns me up. Being with me is like dating a therapist. No, just a healthy woman. I'm confrontational, straight. I don't play any games. Men grow a lot with me. It's like they move through a passage of readiness, and then have to graduate and leave."

This is not just an isolated conversation between Sonya and Hannah. So many women have talked about this situation that there must be a larger pattern here. While a man feels enriched and fulfilled from the experience, he may feel shamed in staying with his teacher. He may need to move on to another woman, where he isn't reminded of his one-down position.

As the women at the next table rise to leave, they lean over and say, "Doesn't make any sense, does it?"

Hannah nods, including them in her response. "You know, I used to think I must be the most screwed-up woman. What's wrong with me? Why do I put the energy into fixing them and then have them go off to another woman? Now, I'm beginning to wonder what's wrong with them that they can't handle it."

Laughing, Sonya agrees. "I'm tired of helping men find their way—with another woman. We should put a sign on our backs: Relationship Teachers for Hire!" The howl from the four women spreads out across the restaurant.

Love Him Or Leave Him, But Stop Kvetching

Sometimes the man leaves you when he has learned what he needs to learn. Sometimes he's scared of investing in a relationship. Sometimes he leaves because you just aren't right for what he needs from a woman.

Often, though, you are the one questioning whether you should stay or leave. Is he right for you?

"Having a wonderful guy in your life is only slightly better than not having a wonderful guy in your life," exclaims Carrie, after an exasperating argument with Allen. "Sometimes I think that maybe I should just get out. But when I think about leaving, I think about having to start over with someone new. I know I would just hit the same snags, or different snags, with another man, but snags nonetheless. So I guess the snags I know are better than the ones I don't know."

Carrie prefers to stay with Allen despite her complaints about him. There is a danger here, though. She can feel validated in her complaints about him, but constant complaining is not useful to her or to Allen; it is an unhealthy basis for a relationship.

As a first step, you always need to identify and amend your own part in your relationship problems. Then, you try teaching your partner what you need from him. If there are still serious problems, you might insist on getting outside professional help from a therapist or counselor. If he doesn't agree, or if the therapy isn't successful, you have to make a decision: do you try harder to make it work, or do you say, "Enough. I'm not trying any more"? Not wanting to give up, but nevertheless unhappy, many women remain in a relationship *and* keep complaining. This is decidedly not healthy!

Think back over the need list you wrote for task number six (see Chapter 9). Often, clearly recognizing what you need *from* a man makes it easier to clearly determine whether the man you are with has the potential to give you what you need. This eliminates the self-doubts that cause you to question whether you are asking for too much, or whether you are worthy of what you want from a man.

You need to assess how much effort you've been putting into helping him become more appropriate for you. Most important, are your efforts paying off?

Are you getting enough of what you need from him as a result of your efforts? Blaming yourself for not doing more prevents you from using your intuition to see if he is willing or able to make the changes you need.

If you keep working harder, with little or no change on his part, or no useful feedback from him on how he (and you) can change, there is a message here that you are ignoring. Now it's *your* issue: Why don't you want to see what is in front of you? It doesn't matter if he can't or won't change. If he's not changing, it's clear he isn't giving you what you need.

At that point, you need to stop whining about him. You have two choices. The first is to accept him as he is, with the things you don't like. You learn to do without what you need from him, maybe finding those qualities in your female friends. Choice number two is to get out.

Here are five steps to help you stop kvetching.

1. After you have clearly identified for yourself what you need but aren't getting from him, *teach* him. Do the best you can.

2. Once you acknowledge that he isn't getting it, for whatever reason, *stop teaching*.

3. Suggest a professional teacher; *go for therapy*. If he goes, great. If he doesn't, he doesn't.

4. If he refuses professional help, *stop complaining!*

5. Make your decision: *Accept him as he is or get out.*

Know when to stop trying. Do your best, don't tackle an impossible task, and don't work overtime. Either the problems are something you can live with or they aren't. Do not blame yourself for not being able to fix the relationship; *it takes two to do that.* If you decide to stay, do so with an awareness of the things that will never change in him. If you decide to leave, you may be sad, but at least you will leave with your self-esteem intact.

In *Being Single in a Couples' World: How to Be Happily Single While Looking for Love* (Free Press, 1998), Xavier Amador and Judith Kiersky answer the question of why women are single. "Everyone wants the best partner possible. But how do you draw the line between a quest for the best and the pursuit of an impossible dream? If you find that no one who is available to you measures up to your hopes and expectations, then you have probably crossed that line" (p. 69).

This theme is too frequently presented in self-help books for women: the woman looks for too much in a man, she is too unrealistic, she should fix herself in some way to get or make a man happy to be with her. Certainly every woman wants the best partner possible, but by midlife, you've lived long enough and been single long enough to know the difference between an "impossible dream" and what you need in a man. This type of comment, tucked away in an otherwise good book, makes me angry at the authors and anxious for the women who read it. It also reinforces those internalized messages that it's a woman's job to find and to fix a relationship. In addition, there's no acknowledgment that a man needs to do his work to make himself ready for a good relationship with a woman! There are no distinctions between the realistic differences between men and women in looking for and working on a relationship.

Afterthought About Teaching

There is a difference between teaching and proselytizing. In talking with a man, you can't say your way is better, but you can say your way is what you need. Then, it is up to the man to decide if he wants to incorporate your way into his. If so, it then *becomes* his way, which means he may not do things exactly as you would wish. He is responding to your telling him what you need, and he's doing it in a way that works for him. It's not your way, but if it gets at what you need, keep quiet and accept it!

That's the point in all good teaching. Teach the underlying principles, and the learners will adapt them to their own style. Be prepared that your "student" will try to teach you what he needs. You must be as open to learning from him as you expect him to be in learning from you.

Therapy
For Single Women

I know a woman who has been in individual therapy for 16 years. She started 4 years before her marriage, and continues to go once or twice a week. I jokingly ask, "Why would you ever want to stop?"

She seriously replies, "I don't intend to!"

It seems she and her husband lead fairly separate lives; they have minimal emotional contact. Her therapy has probably helped the marriage survive. He is nurtured through his work and associates; she is nurtured by her therapist.

What Therapy Can And Can't Do

While I question the ethics of therapy as a form of life maintenance, it can be undeniably helpful as a temporary support. It can help you identify and empower you to stop destructive patterns in your relationships. You can learn more about yourself, and you can acquire tools for dealing with others.

However, therapy can become a psychological hazard. For women who want a "significant other," the therapist (male or female) may unfortunately fill that position. In long-term individual therapy, the therapist can become the most important person in a single woman's life, which means she is not tapping the crucial resource of friendships outside of counseling.

Another hazard of therapy is that therapists may be caught in the same societal confusion about single women as you are. If they are older than 35, they also grew up in a society that first stigmatized single women as "old maids," and then glamorized them. Their therapy may reflect one or the other of these stereotypes, without understanding—without helping *you* understand—the full complexity you experience as a midlife single woman, and the ambiguity you live with in not knowing if you'll ever meet an emotionally available man.

Therapists may also believe that if you solve your personal problems, you can be healthy enough for a man. If they have absorbed the societal trance that women need to be married, they may assume the problems that bring you to therapy are related to your being single (especially if that's what you tell them!).

They may not recognize that regardless of how healthy you get, marriageable men may not be available. In fact, the healthier you do get, the more limited you'll find the pool of men who have also worked on their emotional health.

Trusting Your Intuition

Despite these potential hazards, therapy for a single woman can be invaluable. While it can't make you "right" for a relationship, it can teach you to trust your intuition, especially about men. Women often let the message to find a man block their intuition, not noticing real or potential problems with a man. They may create a fantasy about him, ignoring what he is really showing her about himself. They may tell themselves not to believe what they see in him.

Or they may redefine what they see, making him more acceptable than who he really is. Author Anaïs Nin is quoted as having said: "We don't see things [read, men] as they are. We see them as we are." By discounting what they know about a man, women can diminish the problems by saying, "I'll help him change."

Helen kept excusing Lennie for forgetting their dates, or coming two hours late. He said he was "so busy at work." She didn't want to acknowledge how inconsiderate he was to her.

Whether Lennie was busy or not, his repeatedly not remembering a commitment he made to her gives Helen information about him. Instead of trusting herself and talking with him about how she feels when he is consistently late and doesn't call, she distorts her perception, priding herself on being "supportive and understanding" of him.

Growing up, you may well have been taught to distrust yourself about men. How many times have you returned from being with a man you didn't like only to be told, "You didn't give him a chance," or "You jump to conclusions"? How you felt about him was ignored. These messages build up over the years and may result in your discounting your internal signals about men.

Therapy can help you recognize when you give up your perceptions; it can encourage you to trust yourself, to read a man's behavior more realistically. It can challenge the clichés you may automatically be accepting. For example, when you refer to a man who never talks to you as a "strong, silent man," a therapist can have you consider if he's a "strong, silent man" or just a "silent man." Silent may be fine for you, but you don't need to convert his quietness into a strength he may or may not possess.

Often, your intuition "knows" things about a man that your consciousness hasn't yet noticed. Liz, an Always Single professional woman in her late 30s, is telling me about why men are not interested in her.

"I give off signals that I'm not available," she says.

My antennae are raised. "I'm curious about that. Have you met anyone recently who seemed interested in you?"

She thinks for a second, then recounts, "Well, the other night, a friend told me a man who met me at a party called her to see if I would go out with him."

I push her, "So, somehow he didn't notice your 'not-interested/not-available' signals?"

"Well, I, uh . . ."

"You say you are giving off not-interested signals, but that assumes men are sensitive enough to read your messages."

Liz talks more about the man who did call, wondering if she should go out with him. Then she suddenly switches. "I think I'm using this whole thing of this man so I don't have to deal with the more important issues in my life."

Her switching topics is a jolt. "Liz, that doesn't make any sense. You are dealing with this because it has just happened. You didn't make this man call you right now so you wouldn't have to deal with the more important issues in your life." I return to the topic. "Do you want to go out with him or not? What does your intuition tell you about him?"

"He's really creepy. But that's just a first impression; I really should give him a chance. I'm being too judgmental."

"Perhaps, but perhaps not." I'm sure my voice must have softened when I added, "It's really sad that you can't trust yourself."

Liz has a built-in self-blame Geiger counter. Within five minutes, she has attacked herself three times: she's giving off signals to stay away; she's avoiding important issues; and she's not giving a man a chance. By focusing on what she's doing wrong, she prevents herself from recognizing her perceptions. Yet, her intuition is actively at work, for when I push past her well-rehearsed self-blame, Liz *does* know what she thinks: "He's creepy."

Many women have been well trained to blame themselves when there's a problem in meeting or getting along with a man. Therefore, it's really important for therapists to understand some of the unique issues of working with single women.

How A Therapist Can Help

Regardless of the practitioner's theoretical perspective, a good therapist is a good therapist. Yet, some issues are unique in working with single women—issues a female or male therapist may not have considered. If you are already in therapy or are thinking about beginning, you want your therapist to assess at least three areas about you: the complexity of your feelings, your fix-it strategy, and an explanation for why you are single.

The Complexity Of Your Feelings

You want a therapist to help with your personal baggage: that is, your unfinished family business that interferes with your ability to have a good relationship with a man. You want her to comment when you make bad choices or jump to conclusions about men. You want her to believe that you can live a contented life without a man. You also want her to understand your internal longing (if it's there) to be with a man, without implying a pathological basis for your behavior. You don't want her to convince you that you can live well without a man any more than you need to have a man to live well. Therefore, you need her to be able to help you recognize and own your advantages and drawbacks to being single—even if you don't know them yourself.

Abby struggles with this. "It's hard for me to hear a woman talk about how much she wants to get married and not hear her as desperate or whiny—cardinal sins in our society, you know. So it's just as hard to hear me say it. Add to that my understanding of myself as a feminist—a woman who doesn't need a man to be complete. I'm fine and wonderful just the way I am. But . . ."

She stops. Her eyes seem to be changing colors. "Even when you're confident about yourself as a professional, a role model to others, even when you've got great friends and a good life, you can still feel an emptiness."

Abby is not talking about a pathological emptiness. A full life helps, but it doesn't fill this pain of not loving someone and not being loved in return. Knowing that everyone—even those in happy marriages—experiences existential emptiness doesn't make it easier.

President of a nonprofit educational board, Abby is in her mid-50s. Divorced after a brief marriage in her early 20s, remarried, and then widowed at 34, she completed her master's degree in early childhood education just before her 40th birthday. She taught for a few years until chance moved her into an administrative position, from which she rose to her current managerial role. Working in a field that's predominantly female, she is a good role model for younger single women.

"I don't have it all worked out yet, though. I'm sometimes so filled with loneliness, I think my skin will burst. Yet, other times I'm fine without a man. It's odd. I feel best about myself when I'm not in a relationship! I feel more centered. When I'm in a relationship, it's a struggle to maintain my identity. I think I give up too much of myself; men are so intimidated by my intelligence and my independence.

"Yet, when I'm chairing a meeting or in front of a class, I'm very comfortable with my power. I've noticed too, when I'm not with a man, I live a fuller life. I get together with my friends; I do more interesting things. I feel like my life is more creative, more expansive. I get much more accomplished when I'm not with a man."

Is Abby weak or strong? Does she have a problem that needs therapy? Abby reflects the complex feelings of most competent single women. She needs support and validation that her longing for a man and her emptiness are normal, even for feminists. It would be helpful if she knew that many women feel more centered when not in a relationship.

If Abby were in a relationship, her therapy could help her work on maintaining her full life. Since she isn't, her therapy can help her own the full range of her feelings: embracing both the good things about being single and the drawbacks in not being with a partner. The bottom line needs to be taking control of her life so she has a comfort level with or without a man, and no self-blame for whichever life position she has—for however long she has it.

Your Fix-It Strategy

You want a therapist who recognizes when your presenting problem is an attempted solution to finding a man (see Chapter 3). The fix-it strategy holds that if you can identify a problem that is causing you to be single, and you can fix it, you will be able to find a partner. This strategy is directly related to those old messages about finding a man and about a woman's being responsible for fixing relationships.

Catherine worries that she is frigid; she has no sexual arousal with Peter, a new man in her life. She hasn't had an orgasm with him. I say, "Tell me about this man with whom you are frigid." As she describes Peter, it is clear that he has great difficulty in expressing affection, in sharing feelings, and in enjoying emotional intimacy with her.

I ask if she thinks her body doesn't know how to function right, or is her body telling her something about her feelings toward this man.

She replies, "I'm frigid, so there must be something wrong with me."

I share an old adage: "A woman's body goes on strike if it doesn't like the working conditions."

Catherine doesn't smile. She is giving this serious thought. "You know, I have been orgasmic with other men. I never thought about that."

Peter calls Catherine frigid, and she accepts his indictment. She accepts full responsibility for their sexual problems, no questions asked. It's important that a therapist doesn't do the same. If a woman assumes the problem is hers, then she can work on fixing it. If she accepts that the man has a part in the problem, or it's primarily his problem, then she is helpless.

If your therapist hasn't thought about this, don't be shy; start the discussion. You want a therapist who can help you see when you are accepting responsibility that isn't yours. You want her to remind you that it takes two to fix a relationship problem.

An Explanation For Why You Are Single

You want a therapist who is sensitive to a range of possible explanations for why you are single. Your personal problems may not be the only, or even the prime, reason. (Lots of married women have personal problems too.) It could be plain luck: you have not been in the right place at the right moment. It could be statistics: where you happen to live, the number of single men who want to be married (and, more importantly, the number of men who are emotionally available for a healthy relationship) is disproportionate to the number of women who want to be married. You want a therapist who doesn't have a bias, one way or the other: namely, that you *should* be married, or you *should* remain single. Ideally, you want her to believe that you have what you have for however long you have it. And that whatever you have, you are still the same person.

Questions To Ponder About Your Therapy

If you are not already in therapy, how do you go about choosing a therapist? It can be complicated; even understanding the different types of therapy can be confusing. There are psychiatrists, psychologists, social workers, family therapists, professional counselors, pastoral counselors, and psychiatric nurses. All do some variation of psychotherapy. So, choosing someone based on that person's academic degree may be less useful than thinking about the type of therapy the person does. Although I have degrees in social work and psychology, I identify myself as a feminist family therapist. Sometimes, however, regardless of the theoretical orientation, there's an undefinable click, a chemistry, with the therapist that tells you she or he is right for you.

Whatever your therapist's particular discipline, you want her to be thinking about your situation within the larger social context—not just you and your individual problem. The larger social context includes the influences of your family (parents, siblings, grandparents, etc.) and your religious and cultural background. It also includes understanding the racial, political, and gender factors that have influenced women, especially single women. You don't want a therapist who hasn't changed her thinking as social mores have changed. You don't want a therapist biased for or against single women.

How do you know if your therapist is caught in the social bias—of the old stigma *or* the new idealization—about singles? To help you think about it, here are some questions to consider.

1. Does your therapist think being single is a problem?

2. Does your therapist glamorize being single?

3. Can your therapist hear what it is like for you to be single without imposing his or her own images?

4. Does your therapist interpret all problems with men as your issues?

If you have questions about your therapist's perspective or responses to you, trust your gut. Talk about it; even if you are on target, that may not be enough reason to change therapists. It may be quite rewarding for you and your therapist to discuss personal biases about being single and the effect of the larger societal bias on your therapy. On the other hand, if your discussion doesn't prove fruitful, if you continue to feel she doesn't understand and appreciate the complexity of your being single, trust your intuition. Leave and find a therapist with whom you feel a better fit.

Men And Therapy

Over the course of a year, I see many women, like Maddie, who come to therapy depressed and upset at themselves for being single. Many of these women have done enough of their personal growth work that they *could* have a fairly decent relationship—if they could find a man who has done enough of his work.

It should be a major sadness for our society that these women ask the question, "What's wrong with me?" Sure, therapy can help any woman learn more about herself, but these women aren't there to put finishing touches on what they've already learned. They believe they haven't yet learned *enough*. Maybe, they reason, if they do more, they will be able to find an appropriate partner. For some women, it is easier to feel they haven't done enough than to accept a different reality: namely, the more emotionally healthy they become, the more they are going to restrict themselves because there are far fewer men who are as emotionally healthy as they are.

Men aren't knocking on therapists' doors at the same pace as women. They are more hesitant to do their own personal growth work. They are more likely to knock if they are already in a committed relationship. A man may have a strong enough bond with and love his partner enough that he will do *whatever is necessary* to keep from losing her. If that entails therapy, personal changes, self-reflection, he willingly (or grudgingly) pays the price.

If he is *not* in a committed relationship, he may have little incentive to engage in self-reflection or therapy. If a woman wants more from him, he may decide it's easier for him to withdraw and move on.

This distinction between men who are in and those who are not in a committed relationship is important and may help women absolve themselves from some of the self-blame when a relationship ends.

Ironically, when men do come to therapy and do grow from it, they are usually very pleased. As Allen (from Chapters 9 and 13) observed: "You don't know what you don't know. Carrie dragged me here. I knew we had some problems, but I didn't think they were as serious as she did, and I certainly had no way of knowing how much closer to her I could feel."

Allen and Carrie, both in their 40s, had been seeing each other for a while. Allen had left his marriage 10 years before, and later walked out of a 3-year live-in relationship—without his fully understanding what went wrong each time. "I just knew it wasn't right. The pressure to be who they wanted me to be was too much." He didn't see a pattern in the problems he had with his wife, former partner, and now Carrie.

When he met Carrie, he knew something was different. They fell in love quickly, were hoping to plan a life together, but Carrie kept complaining there was a wall between them. Allen had no idea what she was talking about. Arguments ensued, and finally she told him they had to get professional help or break up.

"I would do anything she asks not to lose her," Allen confesses in their first session together. He is a man many single women would love to know. In their therapy, he struggles with how much of himself he is willing to open to Carrie and to himself, how much he wants to try a new way of relating. He doesn't understand that the particular things they argue about are less significant than the way they handle the argument. Carrie feels discounted, unheard. So does he, but he doesn't have words to explain that. Here's his version of one of their ongoing battles.

"Carrie says, 'Talk to me.' And, I talk—sometimes. Other times, I watch TV or read. But even when I talk, she's unhappy. She says I don't talk about important things. Sometimes I just want to scream, 'What do you want?' I'm so confused."

Like many men, Allen initially makes some changes to please Carrie. It takes some time before he can loosen the shackles of his early gender training and make the changes for himself. He cries as he compares the pain he feels at thinking Carrie doesn't appreciate him with the pain he felt from thinking his father didn't value him as a son. He discovers his panic of losing her is similar to the helpless panic he had as a child when his parents fought. He expresses his shame at two failed relationships.

By the end of their therapy, Allen is saying: "I'm awed at how wonderful it feels sharing all this. I assumed I'd want the floor to open and let me drop in, never being able to face Carrie again—or myself. Instead, my heart swelled as she just held my hand, reassuring me of her love. I don't want to be dramatic, but it really is like my heart grew bigger and warmer." Carrie beams.

Being removed from the constraining gender roles is freeing for both men and women. "You know," Allen observes, "I have no role model for being this kind of man. I love my dad; he wasn't mean and he was always there for me. He just didn't know how to talk about feelings or how to show me or my mother or my sisters that he cared for us. I have had to learn how to be a role model for myself."

Men clearly enjoy the benefits of personal growth. Unfortunately, not enough of them actively seek it out, and too many of them actively avoid it. John, whom we also met in Chapter 9, would have had a different life if he had not turned down Roxanne's offer to go to therapy.

In her individual therapy, after she left him, Roxanne is sad. "For years, I tried to get John to go to therapy with me!" Exasperated, she adds: "I begged and pleaded. I finally got fed up and gave up. I want out now. There's only so much I can try. At some point I have to say my effort isn't paying off. To stay, even though I love or used to love him, would be abusive to me. I'd continue to beat my head against the wall and probably tell myself I wasn't doing enough. I have done enough! I've done more than enough. *Now* he says he'd like to try therapy. Well, it's too late. What a shame it took him so long."

Carrie is luckier than Roxanne. (Really, it's Allen who's luckier than John.) When problems became intolerable, she told him it's therapy or the door. He heard her and grudgingly chose therapy. Roxanne also spoke up, but John wasn't listening.

It's a shame that not enough men are listening. They aren't listening to women, nor are they taking advantage of the growing number of resources for them to learn more about themselves and relationships. Today, more than ever before, there are many good books that contain advice to help men understand themselves better. There are workshops specifically for men, as well as several organizations that support the men's movement.

If you are in a relationship that needs help, try to encourage your partner to participate in therapy. Be prepared, however, that you can't make him. If he refuses, it's not your fault. You tried, now stop trying. And stop beating up on yourself about how much more you should have done to help him get help!

Advice To Therapists Working With Single Women

As therapists, we *do* have an obligation to point out personal issues and old baggage that may be related to a woman's being single. We *do* have an obligation to point out that they can live contented and fulfilled lives as single women, without a man. We *do not* have an obligation to offer advice on meeting men. While some women may need that, therapists may be doing it out of their own helplessness, not knowing what else to do to make a woman feel better. We also *do not* have an obligation to begin the therapy by focusing on—and thereby reinforcing—a woman's pronouncement that her symptoms are a cause of her being single. We can get to that *after* first looking at how she might unnecessarily be absorbing the blame.

Usually, there is nothing a therapist can say to make a woman feel better about being single. This is especially true with midlife women. They have read the books; they've done their therapy; they have full lives. Yet, they still want a man, and they want a therapist to help them make that happen. By offering suggestions on finding men or focusing on what may be the client's own fix-it strategy, you may be reinforcing her self-blame and implying there is something else she could be doing to meet appropriate men.

I have found it more useful to talk *first* about the ambiguity of their being single, and the loss of not knowing if they ever will find a man. I validate their emptiness and focus on how they can feel less empty, given that at the moment there is no man in their life.

When appropriate, I redefine why they are so empty. It's not the lack of a man, as they assume. It's because they have devoted more energy to their career and to finding a man than they have to enhancing their female friendships and doing something meaningful with their life.

Using a work analogy, I show how an energetic devotion to a paid job is rewarded with praise, a promotion, a raise. However, an energetic devotion to a woman's socialized job of finding a husband has none of the same rewards. Instead of praise, she receives criticism: she isn't working hard enough or she's working too hard; she's codependent. After all her efforts, she reaps no job satisfaction (a man), nor validation for her efforts (others' praise for trying to find a man or for how well she lives singly amid couples, who are considered the norm). Her lack of results may be read by others as a sign of her personal failure. She too may believe that.

Although you can't make women feel better about being single, you can help them come to peace with the ambiguity. The best tools for working with single women are validating their feelings and using the nine tasks described in this book to identify areas where they are not enriching their lives. I tell women that they may always feel a sadness about being single. But that sadness doesn't have to be debilitating. If it is, there probably is another underlying issue, like not coming to grips with ambiguous loss, or having a gap in one or more of the tasks.

For instance, single women almost always think more about wanting a man when they are having friendship problems. A lack of intimacy with friends makes the absence of a man more poignant. So does not doing anything meaningful with their life—not feeling settled in their home or job. Remember, the bottom point of the single woman's downward spiral is almost always "if only I had a man."

In working with midlife single women, regardless of their presenting problems, I always keep in mind the *potential effect* of those old internalized messages and their self-blame. I also keep in mind the nine tasks as a tool for assessing what else may be underlying their emotional distress. The following two examples demonstrate how to apply these concepts.

Joyce

Joyce is a 39-year-old Always Single woman who has gone with Larry off and on for five years. She knows he's an alcoholic, but she can't imagine leaving him. She's depressed and seeks therapy because she feels like a failure. She can't get him to stop drinking, yet she won't marry him until he does. She is anxious about turning 40 and still being single.

She sighs. "I dread being an old maid, like my father calls his older sister. And my parents are forever on me to get married. If I leave Larry, I'll let them down."

Finally, as if an afterthought, she notes, "Besides, I'm scared to be alone."

Joyce feels trapped. She has tried therapy before and always quits. During her first session, it is obvious she would rather focus on blaming herself for Larry's drinking than on the sexual abuse she suffered as a child. She says she's not ready to face that yet.

What looks like a simple avoidance of sexual abuse becomes a more complex picture when we consider the six other factors that may be holding Joyce to a bad relationship.

- five-year investment
- turning 40
- difficulty meeting men
- fear of being an "old maid," the family shame
- parental disappointment
- fear of being alone, related to sexual abuse

Each of these factors in itself may be enough reason to be wary about saying goodbye to Larry, and this hasn't even taken into consideration that she loves him!

Keeping all of these factors in mind, it's important to find a focus for the therapy that addresses her self-blame for his drinking, but doesn't ask her (yet) to look at leaving him or at her sexual abuse. An underlying theme in all this is her fear of not being able to take care of herself as a single woman; not being able to deal with her parents' disappointment in her for not being married, and not wanting to be alone without a protector.

Consequently, I suggest we choose a goal that is necessary, whether she leaves Larry or not: taking control of her life. If Joyce decides to stay with him, it should be because she chooses to be with him regardless of his drinking, not because she has failed to get him to stop.

Three months later, Joyce is a regular participant in Al-Anon meetings for people involved with alcoholics. She is in a new apartment that has an active community; she has returned to school for job advancement; and she has improved communication with her close female friends. She has informed her parents that she doesn't want them to talk with her about marriage or say anything about her still being single. She no longer blames herself for Larry's drinking. She has made active steps in most of the nine tasks.

One day, in thinking about her progress, she admits: "I still don't want to leave Larry. I don't want to be alone. Oh . . ." She hesitates, has a moment of insight, then continues, "I don't want to sleep alone!"

She has just realized her fear of being alone is related to her sexual abuse; her father used to come into her bedroom at night. At this point, she decides she needs to face the abuse and her fear before she can make a clear decision about Larry.

Given her past history of therapy, if we had started focusing on why she needed to have an alcoholic in her life, or on her sexual abuse, she might have quit again. Instead, we looked at some of the tasks for living a satisfying single life. As she was feeling better about her home, community, work, and friendships, she felt more empowered to tackle the task of family. Again, Larry must wait.

This can be framed another way: Joyce's family problems must be resolved before she can have a good relationship. Most therapists would accept this assessment. But we never could have *started* with the family problems. She needed to take control of other areas of her life—as a single woman—including getting her parents to back off from pressuring her about marriage. Her willingness to face the abuse came, perhaps, from the strength she gained by mastering the other tasks.

Maddie

Maddie presents a different clinical picture. She is a few months shy of 60 when she begins therapy. Using the tasks with her is helpful in a different way. She complains about being depressed and assumes it's because she is single. I ask her why she is depressed now since she has been without a partner for many years.

Without answering that question, Maddie slips into what seems like a comfortable niche. "I've never been able to get close enough to a man because I'm afraid of intimacy."

"Of course," I respond. "Who isn't afraid of intimacy! But the only way to get more comfortable with it is by doing it. You don't have a man you want to be intimate with now, but what about your women friends?"

As it turns out, she has three very close friends, a satisfying friendship network. She is active in her community, and has good relationships with her remaining family, both parents having died within the past five years. As we go over the tasks, it becomes clear that she has a satisfying life, but is faced with the upcoming developmental change of retirement. Maddie has never really considered what she wanted to do as she aged because: "I'm single, and single women, especially those of us without children, don't seem to age. We always keep doing the same things—looking for a man, working, being with our friends. There is no marker for our aging, like blowing out an increasing number of candles on anniversary or children's birthday cakes."

Maddie is right. While lots of people ignore the realities of aging, for single women there's another grating factor: aging alone. If you keep looking toward a future time when you'll meet a man, you might let other opportunities slip by.

I ask, "If you could look into a crystal ball and see that you would never marry, would that make a difference to your life now?"

She hesitates, then answers, "It's my worst nightmare; yet, I'd adjust." She smiles. "I know just what I would do!" Her face is now aglow with excitement.

"I've been thinking about joining the Peace Corps for the past 10 to 15 years. I always hoped to do it with a man. If I go alone, it's as if I'm giving up the hope of ever finding one."

"And if you give up going because you don't have a man?" I ask.

Maddie begins to cry, a soft gentle moan. There is something pleasing about it. I'm curious. When she stops, she says: "It's as if I've just let go of a huge bag

I've been carrying around with me. I'm sorry to see it go, but I feel a lot freer."

A few weeks later, she feels ready to end therapy. She is no longer depressed. She knows what she needs to do now: decide how to enjoy the next phase of her life, as an older woman, with or without a man.

One year later, I get a postcard from a place in South America I can't pronounce. The only words are: "Peace Corps is the best dream of my life. Still no man, but a much wholer me!"

Even without knowing the specific tasks, many women easily manage singlehood. When they do have difficulty, though, the tasks can be a nonthreatening way to see for themselves what is missing from their lives. The intense loneliness and isolation that many single women report can be eased if they have a satisfying life for themselves at work, and with friends and family.

The nine tasks are a way for therapists to help women gauge why they feel good in their lives and what they can do in the areas where they don't—whether or not they have a partner. Their psychological problems need to be addressed, but only if they are genuine problems. Your job as a therapist is to help separate out problems that belong to them and ones they've accepted as a hoped-for solution to being single.

15

A Different View
Of Being Single

"I can be anywhere—sitting in the movie or at a restaurant, walking down the street or at a business meeting—and I'll see a really neat woman with a wedding band. I wonder how she managed to find a husband. What did she do that I haven't?"

Roberta, like so many other single women, is very together. By all rights, she should be with a really nice man. But she isn't, and hasn't been for many years.

"Or," she continues, "I'll see a really pathetic man, and I'll think how unfair it is that he's got someone at home for him at the end of the day, and I don't. I really don't believe there's anything wrong with me, but it's all around me; it seems like everyone's got someone but me."

Marcelle Clement, author of *The Improvised Woman: Single Women Reinventing Single Life* (W. W. Norton, 1999), makes the exact opposite observations, however. Single women are everywhere, and they love talking about the advantages of not having men in their lives.

Both realities are true. There *are* more single women now than ever before, and we are everywhere. Women *are* more explicit about the difficulties of being married and about their disappointment in men. At the same time, while many women (especially Single Agains) *don't* want to be married, they *do* want a committed partner in their lives.

How do we understand these diverse perceptions of single women? Carol Anderson and Susan Stewart, in *Flying Solo: Single Women in Midlife* (W. W. Norton, 1994), offer one explanation. They interviewed many women who wanted a lover but wanted to avoid "the urge to merge" that happens to so many women in relationships with men. Encapsulated relationships, couples being committed to one another but not living together, are becoming a popular option. Whether the couple is together every night but still maintain their own homes, or they have prescribed times to be together, like weekends, the women feel they have the best of both worlds.

Understanding this distinction between wanting to be with a man who is committed to you and wanting to be married is necessary if we are to unravel the confusion about marriage and singlehood, and the mythology about which is better.

Married Is Not Better Than Single

If men weren't an issue, your leading a single life is not at all unpleasant, particularly if you have accomplished the tasks described in these pages. You've taken control of your life, feel grounded, and have the connection and nurturing that is critical for a satisfying life. Your life has passion and meaning.

You have advantages that you may not have had if you were partnered or married. You know you can take care of yourself. You are independent and self-reliant. You have probably devoted a lot of energy to your personal growth and development. It's not surprising that researchers have found single women to be more emotionally and physically healthy than married men, married women, and single men (in that order).

True, there are disadvantages to being single, such as the absence of touch, of making love with a man you adore, of ready companionship. Let's not make light of these disadvantages; for most women, they are definitely a significant loss. However, you are single now. Later, you may be partnered or married. Still later, you may be single again. It's important to make this distinction: You have no control over when an appropriate man will fit in your life, but you do have control over making the life that you have a good one—for however long you have it.

All women—whether married or single—have the same basic needs. These include, among others, a good self-image, close intimate friendships, companionship, satisfying sexual release.

Marriage doesn't necessarily meet these important needs. By being single, you can imagine that if you were married, you would not feel so depressed, lonely, or needy. By being married, though, you can imagine that if freed from a debilitating marriage, you would not feel so depressed, lonely, or needy. In the old movie *Weatherbee,* a married man advises a single man, "If you don't want to be alone, don't get married."

Two married women in their 40s are talking about a single friend of theirs. Martha, who has a healthy relationship with her husband, says, "I think it must be so lonely for her being single."

Priss, who is discontented with her marriage, is surprised. "No way! She's free from having to mommy a grown man, doesn't have to pick up after a sloppy husband, can have the bathroom all to herself. I think she's damn lucky. She's smart choosing to stay single."

What a shame there has to be *any* discussion about which lifestyle is better. Imagine a world where there was no value judgment placed on being single or married. Where being single would truly be seen as one of two equally viable paths through adulthood; a path that everyone travels for some, if not all, of their adult life; a path with unforeseen twists and turns. Imagine a world where people would pay as little attention to whether you were partnered as they do to the length of your fingers.

A Cultural Revolution

Being single is *not* a problem! Yet, the fact that so many women do not wish to be single makes it a social issue; hence, the need for a cultural revolution. If left to your own devices, you probably would find a way (if you already haven't) to get comfortable with the complexity of being single. You'd probably find a way to deal with the ambivalence about the advantages and the drawbacks. You might even arrive at a peaceful place in dealing with the ambiguity of being single—living with the unknown.

Unfortunately, you are not left to your own devices. You have people like Martha and Priss talking about what it is like being single; you have others telling you *how* you should be feeling and *what* you should be doing about your singleness, as if you *should* be doing something. These messages come from people you know and love, as well as from strangers, songs, ads, books—from just about everywhere! They are direct and indirect.

You may know you are getting the messages, or you may not be aware how the messages influence your life. Whether the messages appear to be positive—"It's a wise woman who knows to avoid marriage"—or negative—"You're so pretty; why aren't you married?"—they are unhelpful and intrusive.

Think for a moment: Do you ever feel anger toward the person who makes these comments? Does it bother you to have someone explaining why you have not "found a man"? Does it bother you that someone thinks you are "too choosy" or, conversely, that you are "smart" to remain single? Does it bother you to have someone assume you have control over whether or not to be with a loving, emotionally available man?

It's bad enough hearing these comments; it's even worse feeling compelled to respond to them. Most women find themselves either agreeing that being single is better, or responding with humor, sarcasm, or defensive language, such as in one comment I hear a lot, "No, I've never been married, but I've been divorced twice (or three times, or whatever the number of important relationships you've had)." Many women bemoan, "It's a no-win situation; no matter what I say, it makes me feel worse."

My pipe dream of a value-free life position (we'd have to get a better term than "marital status") certainly won't happen in our lifetime. In *Single Parents by Choice* (Plenum Press, 1992), Naomi Miller paraphrases Hannah Arendt's ideas about the beginning of the women's movement. In Miller's words: "[A] cultural revolution is not merely a change, but a special event that launches a society in a new direction. It disturbs the status quo so that the old beliefs, values, meanings, traditions, and structures are upset and profoundly modified. If this is so, then we are indeed embarked on a cultural revolution" (pp. 7–8).

Single women desperately need a cultural revolution, and the people to lead it are . . . single women! A nonviolent revolution starts slowly, with quiet shifts in values and behaviors. You can practice at least five of these shifts as you take part in the revolution.

Five Revolutionary Steps Toward Change

1. Retire the old messages
2. Refine your image of a midlife single
3. Set doable goals
4. Deal with ambiguity
5. Nudge, don't shove (when it comes to men)

Step #1: Retire The Old Messages

An essential first step is to get rid of the old messages (see Chapters 2 and 4) that no longer fit for you. If you still hold some dear, by all means keep them. But remove the archaic ones and replace them with new messages that are more applicable to who you are today. For instance:

- Be yourself, with or without a man.
- Trust your intuition.
- Be appropriately choosy and fussy.
- Show your smarts. (Accept only a man who can accept who you are.)
- Remember that male egos aren't so fragile.
- Don't defend yourself when asked, "Are you married?" A simple "No" is sufficient.
- Ask yourself: "Do I like him? Is he worthy of my time and effort?"
- Remind yourself that as you get older, you get wiser and better.
- Become the man you wanted to marry.
- Be yourself, with or without a man. (It's worth repeating!)

Reflection: Retiring The Old Messages And Creating New Ones

1. Look back over your own list of messages in Chapter 4.
2. Separate out the ones that no longer fit you today.
3. Think about what type of ritual or "retirement party" you would like to make for these outdated messages. (See Chapter 5 for ideas about creating rituals.)

4. Make a new list of messages you want to live by; make them fit who you are today.

5. Take your time. Keep adding to this list of new messages for being single.

Step #2: Refine Your Image Of A Midlife Single

It's hard to distinguish yourself as an "adult single" because there's no societal demarcation or ritual that differentiates between you as a young single and you now. When did you stop being a young single? Did you or anyone else note your passage into being an adult single? If so, what helped you make that transition? What were the notable differences for you? Most women don't have clear transition markers.

If you have always been single, your lifestyle may not have changed much throughout your adulthood. You know you have personally matured, professionally grown, and lived a life that has influenced who you are today. You may have more money, own property, follow the stock market, but others may still see you as they did when you were younger. You don't have the "markings"—that is, a husband and children—of a woman whose life has changed.

If you are returning to singlehood, your last prior experience as a single may have been as a young adult. You don't want to return to being single with that as your image. There should be significant differences between you as a young single and you as an adult single.

Imagine . . .

> You were at an event the other night and met a potentially interesting man. You had a delightful time with him and noted his saying at various points in your conversation, "We'll have to go canoeing sometime," and, "You've never been to the opera? I'll have to take you." He certainly sounded interested in you and spoke as if he intended to be seeing lots more of you. Now, here it is, eight days later, and you still haven't heard from him. Much to your dismay, you find yourself hoping he's on the other end of your ringing telephone.

Did this happen 20 years ago or this year? Many women are 20 years older but are still responding with the same behaviors: still waiting for a man to call; still wondering if he's interested in them. Similarly, many single men are 20 years older but still acting like they did just out of college, pressuring women for sex, playing hard to get, promising a future together, then disappearing.

Times have changed. You have maturity on your side. Twenty years ago you had to wait for him to call. Today, if *you* are interested in seeing *him* again (making this distinction is another indication of your maturity), you can call him to get closure. Waiting for a man to call leaves you hanging.

You want to know, Does he or doesn't he want to get together? If he does, maybe he doesn't call because he is shy or busy. If you call him, though, and he quickly ushers you off the phone, you've got your answer: he's not interested. It's a clear sign you should forget him, spend no more time thinking about him.

You can express an interest in a man, but there's no point in chasing after him. If he doesn't want to be with you, if he can't show you he's interested in being with you, that's a clear sign he can't give you what you need—to be wanted by him!

There's something else that should also be different by virtue of your being older and wiser—your language. Eighteen-year-olds go on "dates" with their "boyfriends." Midlife women should have a more appropriate language for what they do, and with whom.

Without thinking about yourself as an adult single, you may be perpetuating behaviors based on the only role model you have—yourself as a young single. Part of taking control of your life is deciding what type of adult single you want to be, and then setting doable goals for yourself.

Step #3: Set Doable Goals

For women whose goal is to be married or partnered, you may be setting yourselves up for failure because a good marriage is not necessarily within your control. You can *want* to be married, but to achieve that requires more than perseverance. Despite all of your efforts, you have no control over making an appropriate man appear. Therefore, a goal of marriage may leave you perpetually feeling unsuccessful and like a failure.

After a year of therapy, Patty had made considerable gains. She was no longer depressed; was clearer about what she needs from a man; separated herself from her parents' expectations for her; changed to a more personally gratifying career. She was immensely happier than she had ever been. She felt grounded in her home, work, and social life.

One day, though, she admitted: "I can really see how much I have changed. I know I feel healthier and better within myself. But I'm not any closer to my goal."

"Which is?" I ask.

"Being married. I'd willingly give up all these changes if that would help me get married."

Regardless of her accomplishments, Patty's primary goal is to be married. Without that, she feels unsuccessful. The goal she has set for herself, however, is an unattainable one since it isn't within her power to bring an emotionally available man into her life. Patty resented letting go of her goal of marriage, but over time, she reluctantly made a list of more doable and self-enhancing goals.

- Make my life as meaningful as possible, whether or not I marry.

- Carefully choose when and where I go to meet men, and go only when I want to.

- Be choosy. Remind myself that I am worthy of an *appropriate* man, not just any man. I cannot *make* him appear.
- Believe that I am just as worthy a person if I am married or single.
- Gently, firmly, and consistently stop my parents from making comments about me and men.

Reflection: Changing Undoable To Doable Goals

1. Take nine index cards and label each with one of the tasks described in Chapters 4 through 12.
2. For each task, list specific goals you want to set. Be concrete and realistic.
3. Get a second opinion: share your goals with a good friend and ask if they seem within your control.
4. For any goals you listed that aren't within your control, think about why you thought they might be. (Were you influenced by some of the old messages?)

Reflection: More About Doable Goals

1. List 25 things you want to do before you die. They may be major (like traveling through Egypt by camel) or minor (like sitting at a cafe and sketching passersby).
2. If you have trouble coming up with 25, keep the list in sight so you can add to it. You should want to do more than 25 things in your remaining years!
3. Check each one off as you do it. Periodically assess your progress. There's no particular rush, since you have until you die, but you do want to make sure you're working on your special list.

Step #4: Deal With Ambiguity

Sherri, one of the several women in my study who said they had "never been married but had been divorced twice," made this observation. "If you have a good relationship with a man, you can get on with the rest of your life. If you don't want a relationship with a man, you can get on with the rest of your life. But if you don't have a relationship, and you want one, trying to find it *becomes* the rest of your life."

Our cultural revolution must provide strategies to prevent this from happening. If Sherri were to label her feelings as ambiguous loss (not knowing if she will ever find an appropriate man), trying to find a man might not become the rest of her life. Pauline Boss identifies five strategies for dealing with ambiguous loss in medical and life crises in her chapter of *Living Beyond Loss,* which was mentioned in a different context in Chapter 10. These can likewise be adapted for single women's ambiguous loss.

The first strategy is *labeling ambiguity as a major stressor.* "Just having the situation labeled by a professional as ambiguous and hearing empathy for that dilemma helps [people] to withstand a lack of clarity . . . [and] to cope with it" (pp. 168–69). For many women, this alone helps them reverse a pattern of internalizing feelings of responsibility, blame, shame, and failure.

The second strategy is *talking with family and friends* to exchange feelings and to learn to tolerate different perceptions. For example, a daughter would hear and understand her parents' wish for her to be married, while they simultaneously understand how she feels when they keep asking her about men.

The next strategy is *assessing your efforts to find a man.* If you are satisfied with what you have done to meet men (and are not swayed by an internal message to try harder), then even if you are unsuccessful, you can validate your efforts. Give yourself credit for what you have been doing.

The fourth strategy is social interaction, *talking with other singles.* This does not mean complaining to each other about men, which many single women do. As part of the cultural revolution, the talking must grapple with how to remove self-blame, how to deal with the social pressures, how to dismantle the old messages. This talking breaks the isolation among women and stimulates ideas for contending with those who unwittingly perpetuate the stigma against singles, including themselves. This type of talking may be done informally with your friends, or you may find—or start—a support group for midlife single women.

Finally, *finding some positive meaning in your being single—right now—is important.* Without being a Pollyanna, you can identify how you have emotionally grown, or things you have done that may not have been possible if you had been partnered. For Single Again women, consider what you have learned and done since you've been without a husband. Finding positive meaning in your singleness does not remove your wish (if you have one) to be married; it does not remove the hope that marriage might still happen. It merely validates that you have not been wasting your time without a man.

For women who want to be with an appropriate partner, it is understandable that they feel an ongoing pain for what they can't have. No one—family, friends, therapists, you, yourself—should talk you out of the sadness of that loss. What you can do, nevertheless, is remove the self-blame; it may not be your fault. Then, while you are still left with the sadness, you can learn to live with the ambiguity of not knowing if you ever will meet an emotionally available man by applying the five strategies above. (Chapter 10 offers still more ideas for doing just that.)

Five Strategies For Dealing With The Ambiguous Loss Of Being Single

1. Labeling ambiguity as a major stressor

2. Talking with family and friends about your being single, listening to their feelings about your being single, and learning to tolerate each other's different perceptions

3. Assessing and validating your efforts to find a man

4. Talking with other women about contending with the social prejudice against singles

5. Finding some positive meaning in your being single—right now

Step #5: Nudge, Don't Shove

In the early years of discussing gender inequality in organizations, one particular professional mental health association was being ripped apart by the tension. The women were angry that the male leadership discounted them, and were challenging the men to give them greater participation. The men didn't believe they excluded the women, and they were angry at being unfairly attacked.

At the association's annual convention, the men ignored the women, complained to each other, and talked of dropping out. The women met together to talk about how we felt left out, how to strengthen our role in the organization, and how to increase our connection with each other. (This parallels what I see in my office: It's the woman who wants to shift the power imbalance in the relationship, and the man's reaction is to pull away emotionally or physically.)

From that meeting came the novel (at the time) idea of initiating a women's-only session for the next year's convention. Caught up in the excitement and powerful potential of this same-sex meeting, I suggested we tell the men what we were doing; they might want to have their own men's meeting. There was loud opposition. "There we go again; taking care of men." "That's their problem." "We can't do it for them. They have to take care of their own needs."

While I wholeheartedly agreed with the comments, I knew the men would probably never think about joining together to deal with their complaints about the women or about re-balancing the structure of the organization. For the sake of the association, we needed to nudge them. We couldn't wait for them to think on their own about the value of having such a meeting.

Despite criticism from some women, I approached one man. I told him what the women were going to do the following year and suggested he think about the men doing the same. His initial response was great idea, but no thanks. I gently insisted he just *think* about it. He might choose not to do anything, but at least he shouldn't ignore the idea. He walked away slightly annoyed.

The next afternoon he caught up with me on the escalator and matter-of-factly reported that "the first Men's Group Planning Committee" had been established and had met that morning! More than a decade later, this group is still highly popular. In fact, some men come to the conference primarily for the men's meeting.

Olga Silverstein, a well-known feminist family therapist who has written about mothers and sons in *The Courage to Raise Good Men* (Viking, 1994), believes that women understand men better and more readily than men do themselves. Since we relate so well with men, it seems reasonable for us to use our understanding to open a door for men—or at least point out there is a door—but not shove them through it.

It's a shame men's therapy and support groups have not become more socially acceptable. I have run many of them over the years, and men *do* enjoy talking to each other, sharing feelings, and supporting each other's growth. They just don't know they enjoy it until they are doing it. The real challenge is to nudge just enough to get them to the first group session.

If men don't get emotionally healthier, women lose. But women can't do it for them; men must find their own growth paths. It's in your benefit to help a man make changes, to grow emotionally, as long as

• you want to.

• it isn't at your own expense.

• you see results to warrant your efforts, and you stop when you don't.

• you don't feel responsible if he decides not to make any changes.

Teaching him doesn't mean that you haven't contributed to the communication problems, or that there is nothing you can learn from him. It just means that someone has to get the learning ball rolling, and if it isn't you, it might never get rolling.

Use Your Anger To Mobilize The Revolution

People pushing for a cultural revolution are often the brunt of name calling. I've been labeled an "angry man hater." Man hater? Absolutely not. Angry? Yes. I am angry, at men in general—they aren't doing enough to improve their emotional selves. They don't seem to be bothered by the condescending cartoons, contemporary cards, and jokes that attack their lack of sensitivity. When I showed men from my single men's study contemporary cards that derided men, they laughed and either agreed with the comments or discounted them.

Change comes when there is enough discomfort and passion to mobilize people. Contrary to women of 35 years ago who rebelled against "woman bashing," men don't get indignant at how they are perceived. In the 1970s, women pulled together to fight back; they started consciousness-raising groups; they became politically active. As a result, the women's movement has opened the doors to more dramatic changes than the men's movement—which started around the same time.

Why not? Maybe men aren't bothered because women haven't told them that there's a problem. Maybe they aren't bothered because they have "toughened up" in order to "become a man." Maybe they are used to sarcasm as a form of jesting with each other.

Decades ago, women didn't like the condescending attitudes toward us. We didn't like being second-class citizens, so we did something about it. We struck back against traditional female socialization that prevented us from growing to our full potential.

Men, as a whole, haven't begun to look at how they have been handicapped by their socialization. Fortunately, many individual men *are* bothered enough to want to change. Unfortunately, though, they're not as successful in mobilizing others as women have been. Not enough men are looking to change the larger social picture of how they have been socialized as males. As a group, men are not worried enough about protecting future generations of little boys from the messages *they* were taught.

Some of you reading this will disagree and want to argue with me about these ideas. Don't. Let the men do that. They're the ones who should be reacting. Let them write their own books about Clues for Understanding Women Better, Emotionally Available Women, What Men Need from Women (see Chapter 9). Let them *buy* the books that are already written by and for men. Let men charge into activism and empower the men's movement. I'm more interested in having men arguing about these issues. Women spin our wheels arguing with each other when the only real change can come from men.

Yes, I am angry. I am angry that women protect men from our anger. I'm angry that so many women blame themselves for being single instead of blaming the dearth of emotionally available men. I'm angry that our society gives lip service, not genuine effort, to removing the value judgment that it's better to be married than to be single.

I'm not afraid of my anger; don't be afraid of yours. Anger is empowering. (See Harriet Lerner's *The Dance of Anger* [Harper & Row, 1985] for constructive ways to use your anger.) Change comes when people are mobilized and empowered by their anger, when they take action and encourage others to take action. Being angry is not the same as being bitter or nasty or cruel. Being angry is a strength that propels others to use their strength, that can eventually bring about a socially needed change.

Mobilizing The Revolution On Two Fronts

She's only 35, but she has an enviable maturity. As she walks toward the chair, Brenda's long gray knit dress and jacket accentuate her height and poise. Though secure at work, Brenda is, unfortunately, shaky when it comes to dealing with men.

"I've been thinking about what you said last week. If I believe you, then I'm angry."

"*If* you believe me?"

"Well, you said my not meeting a man wasn't because there's something wrong with me."

"Right." We had spent weeks looking at her part in why prior relationships hadn't worked and at the men she had been meeting.

"But other people think it's me. My parents blame me. (Pause) I told you, there were only two men in the past two years that I was at all interested in. The first one I dated for a while, but it became clear he had a serious drinking problem."

"You used good discretion in getting out," I validate.

"The second one was just a few months ago. I *know* he, we, both of us, had a good time. We were just to meet for coffee, but he suggested extending it to dinner and then later to ice cream too. We had a wonderful conversation. We had so much in common; we even talked about how some men are intimidated by strong competent woman. He said he wasn't and couldn't understand why other men were. Then I never heard from him again. I dropped him an e-mail, but no response."

"What do you think happened?"

"My first impulse is to say I must have been wrong; he didn't enjoy it as much as I thought. But after hearing you last week, I'm questioning that. Unless he was a great con artist, I know he enjoyed being with me. Maybe he's learned how to mouth all the right words about liking strong women, but he was really scared of me. Maybe he has a girlfriend, or he's gay. Who knows!

"I've been thinking all week about what it means if I don't take responsibility for not meeting men I want to be with. That would really underscore how few men there are to choose from. That would limit my choices, and *that* would make me angry!"

I nod. This is always painful; giving up self-blame initially leaves women feeling worse. Without self-blame, they really are not in control of the absence of having a partner. Encouragingly, I offer: "When you blame yourself, you turn your anger inward. Far better you should be angry at society, men in general, or a specific man for not being emotionally healthy enough to have a relationship with you."

"In my gut, I know you're right, but this goes against everything I've always heard." Her voice trails off. After a brief pause, Brenda resumes. "What do I say to my parents, my married friends, my single friends? It's like being at the start of a revolution that no one wants, so no one wants to enlist."

A few weeks later, Brenda walks into the office, seeming a bit taller. She sits down and starts in right away, as if we are in the middle of a conversation.

"Okay. I accept the premise it's not me; I know in my gut this is true. I really do have much—not all, but much—of my stuff together. I'm not so afraid of intimacy that I would mess things up without knowing I was doing it. Besides, I'm not even meeting men to have a chance to mess things up with!

"So, I've decided," she asserts, with the same poise she uses at work, "I'm not afraid of my anger. I want my mother, my friends, everyone to stop blaming me or implying I could be doing something about being single. What can I do?"

As with all cultural revolutions, you need to know what needs changing, and you need a plan. Single women are confronted constantly with biases, stereotypes, and nonsensical messages from society, in general, and from close family and friends, in particular. This situation needs to be changed. While you may not want to take on the world, it is crucial for you to at least notice each incidence of being faced with one of the belittling messages or stereotypes. Then decide for yourself how, when, or if you want to speak up.

You may prefer to make changes only within yourself. You may want to confront the biases and messages you hear from others—some of the time or all of the time. Not saying anything, though, is different from not noticing. You *always* need to notice the messages. The two arenas, then, for confronting the messages are within yourself and within society.

Confronting The Messages Within Yourself

Whether through self-help books, therapy, or women's consciousness-raising groups, the primary arena for confronting the old messages is yourself, your own internalized biases. Only after you recognize how you buy into self-blame and heed the messages can you begin to stop others from inflicting them on you and to stop yourself from inflicting them on other single women.

Do you notice when your friends chide you for not liking a man you just met or for "not giving him a chance"? Do you notice when you do it to them? Do you notice the connection between feeling sorry for yourself for being single and having just heard a romantic song or seen a commercial that implies being a couple is the valued norm?

The message that being single is not as valued as being married is so pervasive and subtle, it can be hard to see. You might spend a week or so with a notebook, jotting down each time you see, hear, say, or feel something that diminishes you as a single woman. At first you may not even know what you are looking for.

With practice, though, you may begin to notice that most commercials imply you are missing the American dream of being a couple in all aspects of your life—from buying a car, to smoking a cigarette, to shampooing your hair, to getting stains out of dirty shirts. If you live in a commuter-dependent city, you may notice that the Kiss and Ride signs you used to think were cute are really a message of exclusion. And, more directly, how often do you hear statements from friends, or even strangers, indicating you should be married, or you are less adult because you are single?

You may find yourself feeling depressed as your list grows. Don't de-press your feelings, turning against yourself. Instead, think how you can mobilize your anger in a way that is consistent with your personality and lifestyle. Depression can be anger turned inward, while anger can be personally empowering.

Here are five ideas for empowering yourself while countering the biases against your being single.

No Excuses

When asked if you are married, a simple answer of "No" suffices; no apologetic or defensive jokes are necessary. Although a clever response may make you feel better at the moment, it carries with it the underlying message "I have to have some excuse for remaining single." You don't need any excuse, however; your singleness is just a statement of fact.

Establish Your Role(s) In Life

Part of the discomfort of being single is the lack of an established or positive role for "non-wives" and "non-mothers." In some parts of South America, a single woman has the honored role of being the *uanaa,* the professional chaperon. In North America, a single woman just plays the outdated and pejorative role of the "maiden aunt." Therefore, empower yourself by figuring out what roles are most special to you. This supports the fifth strategy for dealing with ambiguous loss, finding some meaning or benefit in your being single (as described in Chapter 10).

For myself, because I am single, I have more time and energy to devote to my personal roles of daughter, sister, aunt, and friend. In my professional world, by virtue of being single, I bring a unique perspective to my valued roles as therapist, teacher, and mentor.

You may be saying, "Big deal; so she's a daughter, sister, blah, blah, blah." As women, we tend to diminish the importance of these roles, yet they really are special, and we shouldn't take them for granted. By diminishing the importance of your roles, you diminish the difference you make to those who give you the identity—your parents, your siblings, your nieces and nephews, your friends, your students, your customers or clients, etc.

Find a Balance Between Hope For The Future And Enjoyment Of The Present

The women in my study were clear; they *want* to keep hoping they will eventually meet an appropriate partner. Maintaining the hope keeps them feeling sensually vital and wards off emptiness. However, while finding a way to live with the ambiguity of not knowing if the future holds a man for you, it's also important to balance the hope with an appreciation for the life you have in the present. Some single women are still so focused on the future, "when I meet him," that they forgo the full pleasure they could be having in their daily experiences.

Before you quickly dismiss this, saying, "that's not me," remember that this focus on the future can carry over to other aspects of your life besides men. Does the following example sound familiar?

You are driving on a back road and see an antique shop, a fruit stand, a calf and its mother—whatever. You feel the impulse to stop, but you keep going, telling yourself it isn't necessary, you don't need anything, you are in a hurry, the car behind will get upset, there is no place to turn around, etc. All of these may be true, but when such responses become routine, that is, when you *always* pass something by because it is easier than stopping, you have lost the importance of the present.

Empower yourself; every aspect of your life can be important and significant—*to you!* With or without a man, enhance your life. The present makes your life more meaningful.

Identify What Gives Your Life Meaning

Ask yourself this question: "If I were happily married, with 2.3 healthy children, and I was told I had to have something else of importance in my life, what would it be?"

Ask yourself the crystal ball question: "If you could see that you would meet a wonderful man, but not for 5, 10, or 15 years, how would you live your life now?"

You need to feel that your existence matters—not just to a man, but in the world. When you are 99 years old, what will you feel proud about as you reflect upon your life? What did you contribute to society that had even some tiny significance? What did you do with your years that filled you with a passion?

Investing time in a community organization or a charity because you are a helpful and kind person is not the same as doing it because you feel passionately about contributing to a greater good, or making the world more beautiful or friendly.

Making your life more meaningful does not mean contributing your time and energy without any reward. You should feel some benefit from your giving, but are you giving a lot to others and getting little back from them? The reward may be concrete, such as being thanked and appreciated, or spiritual, or just knowing you are making a difference in the world. The reward is in the way you feel about yourself as a result of giving to others. The mutuality of the giving and receiving adds to your self-image, your self-esteem, and your self-identity. This is true when you are giving to a man, a friend, an organization, or any good cause.

Identify What You Need From (Not In) A Man

Those old messages about men didn't include thinking about your needs. Fortunately, many women today are more aware of their needs. However, they often think of what they need *in* a man, such as personality traits, interests, values. Instead, empower yourself by considering what you want *from* him, *for* yourself. This is different from what you want him to be like.

Instead of saying you want him to be sensitive, for instance, you might say you want a man who can be sensitive to you. Instead of wanting him to be intelligent, you want a man who can converse with you and who is interested in what you have to say. This is more than mental gymnastics. The underlying point is very different: it's not what he can give you; it's what you need from him. The emphasis is on your taking control of identifying your needs.

There's another issue you should consider. Research shows that one of the more significant factors in healthy, long-lasting relationships is the partners' support of one another in their growth and change. Therefore, you might include on your list wanting a man to allow you room to grow personally and professionally. You don't want him to be threatened by your changes. In addition, you may want him to actively encourage your own growth and maybe even undertake his own.

Periodically Check How You Are Doing On The Tasks

The nine tasks described in Chapters 4 through 12 can help you confront the old internalized messages and remind you how well you are doing as an adult single. You probably aren't perfect in all tasks; there may be some where you are doing quite well and some where you notice some deficits. When the pull from the old messages makes you feel bad about being single, this is the time to pay attention to the deficit areas. Shifting your focus from feeling bad about being single to enhancing your life as a single does not mean you are committed to being single. It simply means you are committed to living the best life you have at the moment.

Another way to use the tasks is to see where you experience the most pain in your life and then reread that chapter. You may well find clues for the causes and the cure.

A third way to use the tasks, especially on days when you feel blue, is to focus on all that you have accomplished, reminding yourself of the strength you possess in being an adult single in a world that values married couples.

Confronting Messages Within Society

Some women become angry when they begin to see all the cultural biases against singles. If this happens to you, be sure to use your anger productively, channeling it in ways that make you feel good, that serve some larger purpose. Don't just vent steam everywhere, for you'll be called (and may feel like) a bitter woman.

The message that being single is not as valued as being married exists on an institutional level and on a community level, as well as among the people in your life. Therefore, each time you hear a comment or a message that belittles singles, you need to decide if you want to respond, and if so, on which level.

For instance, on an institutional level, if an advertisement on television or in a magazine offends you as a single woman, you may want to start a petition noting your complaint. Then, send the petition to the marketing division of the product's manufacturer, as well as to the media that carry the ad. Each time you hear the media call a single woman "unmarried," you can decide if you want to write a letter pointing out the absurdity of defining a woman by what she is not.

On a community level, decide if you want to say anything when you are stuck in the back corner of the restaurant at a table for one. Or if you want to take on your country club that admits only married men and their wives, excluding Always Single and Single Again women. You choose whether or not to speak up if your synagogue or church has religious services and rituals that are not inclusive—addressing the needs of both singles and families. (Sponsoring services and rituals exclusively for singles is considerate, but this separation makes a distinction between being a single and a married adult.)

On an individual level, you have the same choices with the people you know: either speaking up or not when you hear messages and biases about singles. Do you say anything when the store clerk—a man 20 years your junior—calls you a "young woman" or a colleague calls you a "girl"? While they probably say this to married women too, when you hear it as a single, it reinforces the old message that you are not yet an adult. "Young woman" and "girl" are demeaning terms that imply you need someone to take care of you.

Is being so literal with our language making too big a deal about nothing? That same question was asked 40 years ago when some Southerners called African American men "boys." Cultural revolutions require attention to prejudicial language.

You need to *hear* any messages from your family that indicate they see you as less adult because you are single—whether or not you choose to respond. If you do respond, be sure to do so without rancor. If you want to teach them to talk differently with you, you need to be forthright and kind. For instance, when your mother asks why you don't go out with a particular man, you might remind her, without sarcasm, that you are qualified to make important decisions all day, so she should trust you to have used your same good judgment in this decision.

When your siblings and their spouses get together socially, you might want to question why they invite you only when there is a man in your life. Your family may not change their attitude or belief about singles, but they can change their behavior and words when they are around you!

If you are angry at how others talk to you or treat you, remember that you can choose how to respond to them. For families, adjusting to new ideas is often difficult (as we discussed in Chapter 11). Attaching these new ideas to verbal attacks, sarcasm, and nastiness is guaranteed to be counterproductive. Always use kindness and, whenever possible, try humor.

Deciding when and how to respond to the messages and biases about singles gives you some sense of control over a situation (that is, not having a partner) that is out of your control. Keep in mind that no one intentionally is out to be mean or unfair to single women. Everyone has been raised with the same destructive messages. Reeducation is necessary for us all, and the best teachers are those who are most affected—single women.

Single Pride

The nine tasks are a good gauge of your comfort level in living a satisfying single life. When you take control of your life, you feel emotionally connected to others; you feel nurtured and nurturing—with or without a man.

You have *met your basic needs* for daily contact, security, physical touch, rituals, and meaningfulness in life. You *feel grounded* in a home that reflects who you are, and in your neighborhood. You spend your days at a gratifying job, and you have a satisfying social life. You *enjoy intimacy* with close friends who can add to your personal and professional growth. You have *made a decision about the role of children in your life,* accepting what is, changing what you want, and grieving what can't be. You have *faced your sexual feelings,* finding a balance between acknowledging and distracting them.

You have *clarified your thinking about men,* becoming bilingual, communicating with them better, and identifying what you need from a man. You have *grieved* your lost dreams, accepted the ambiguity about being single, and separated out your grief from others'. You have *made peace with your parents,* honoring the positives you have gotten from them and dropping the negatives. You have *prepared for old age,* thinking about what identity you want as an older woman, improving relationships with those you will want in your life then, and attending to your financial and legal affairs.

When you are old and look back over your life, you know you will feel content with what you have done with what you have had. I have an Always

Single male friend in London who talks about "solo pride." With his permission, I amend his phrase to "single pride." He's got part of it right. You certainly should feel proud about how well you take care of yourself; you should feel pride in having an enriched life in a world that is not designed for single women. But you definitely can't do it solo; you need people. That is an underlying principle of the nine tasks: you need to be connected with others; you need the mutuality of nurturing and being nurtured.

The following anonymously came across the Internet. Written for all women, I have adapted it specifically for single women.

As part of Single Pride, every single woman should have

- one old love who reminds her how far she has come.
- a childhood she's content to leave behind.
- a past juicy enough that she's looking forward to retelling it in her old age.
- the realization that she is actually going to have an old age and some money set aside to fund it.
- one friend who always makes her laugh and one who lets her cry.
- a good piece of furniture not previously owned by anyone else in her family.
- eight matching plates, wine glasses with stems, and a recipe for a meal that will make her guests feel honored.
- a set of screwdrivers, a cordless drill, and a black lace bra.

As part of Single Pride, every single woman should know

- how to fall in love without losing herself.
- how to quit a job, break up with a lover, and confront a friend without ruining the friendship.
- when to try harder and when to walk away.
- how to ask for what she wants in a way that increases her chances of getting it.
- that she can't change the length of her calves, the width of her hips, or the nature of her parents.
- that her childhood may not have been perfect, but it's over.
- where to go when her soul needs soothing—be it her best friend's kitchen table or a charming country inn.

Single Pride does not mean it is better to be single than married; it simply means that you are taking control of your life, whatever it is at the moment—with or without a man.

Afterword:
A Personal Note

During the time I was writing *With or Without a Man,* my life took many twists and turns. Those years fully confirmed that real life happens, whether you are married or single. My father became ill and died. My mother became ill and survived. My dog died. My favorite uncle became ill, survived, and then was killed a few months later. A very close female friend pruned me from her friendship garden—with no explanation. I made two new close friends. I was involved in a potentially serious relationship which ended. I gave myself a fantastic 50th birthday weekend event. My siblings and their children and I started a yearly get-together, just for us. My clinical practice kept growing, and I published a few other books.

Many good things and many painful ones.

Sometimes, not always, it was a struggle facing the difficult periods without a life partner. My closest friends, though, were an incredible support. And rereading segments of the manuscript offered clarity when I felt overwhelmed and couldn't distinguish between what was appropriate grief and what was downward spiraling. The nine tasks proved a guideline for me, personally, to see how I was doing. They pinpointed where I was stuck and when I blamed that impasse on being single. It was also a real eye-opener, as I read over the chapters again, to recall which ones were the most difficult to write. I can only assume that they were the tasks that still needed more of my own attention.

Further Reading

Anderson, Carol, and Susan Stewart. *Flying Solo* (W. W. Norton, 1995).

Bravo! A long-overdue book. Using the theme of flying an airplane, the authors found that once single women have given up the dream of the prince, they triumph in flying solo. Anderson and Stewart interviewed 90 Always Single and Single Again women between the ages of 40 and 55 and who have lived on their own for at least a number of years. They found these women are successful in being single; that is, they are upbeat and positive. Of particular note are the fresh ideas about the role of work for single women, and encapsulated relationships.

Erickson, Beth. *Longing for Dad: Father Loss and Its Impact* (Health Communications, 1998).

The cover is great and so are the personal and professional stories inside. This is about growing up without a father present—physically or emotionally. Of particular interest is the chapter on the seven sources of father hunger. This is useful for women who want more understanding of the effect of this loss on their relationships with men. The book is sprinkled with helpful action exercises.

Friday, Nancy. *My Secret Garden* (Pocketbooks, 1973).

This book is in its 25th edition, which obviously means women continue to read it. If you can't find a copy, keep looking; it is worth the effort. For women who have difficulty generating their own sexual fantasies (for masturbation and for lovemaking), this is a treasure trove.

Imber-Black, Evan, and Janine Roberts. *Rituals for Our Times* (Harper Collins, 1992).

If the idea of rituals grabs your attention, grab this book. Part Two explains how to set them up, and Part Three gives hundreds of ideas for including rituals in your daily life, for special events, holidays, vacations, and lots more.

Isaacs, Florence. *Toxic Friends, True Friends* (Morrow, 1999).

Given the importance of friends for women as you move through midlife and into old age, this book is a must. It confirms feelings you've had about friends but couldn't explain. One chapter is devoted specifically to single women and friends, one to friends after a divorce, and one to friendships with siblings.

Lerner, Harriet. *The Dance of Anger* (Harper & Row, 1985).

Although this book is 15 years old, it should be a dog-eared addition to your nightstand. Women constantly need to be reminded how empowering anger can be—when it is used well. Whether with men, bosses, or coworkers, parents or friends, there are patterns of moves and countermoves that can prevent you from being derailed in expressing your anger effectively.

Osherson, Sam. *Wrestling with Love: How Men Struggle with Intimacy* (Fawcett, 1992).

Yes, this is a book for men, but it's helpful for women to understand that men are lonely for relationships and eager for connection. It explains how shame and anger distort feelings of intimacy—with the women in their lives, their children, their parents, and their friends. If you could just pass this along to every man you know—*and make sure he reads it*—there'd be a lot more emotionally available men out there for single women.

Pogrebin, Letty Cottin. *Among Friends: Who We Like, Why We Like Them, and What We Do With Them* (McGraw-Hill, 1987).

This is a wonderful old book on friendships. It covers different levels of friends, both at work and in personal life, fights and resolutions, men's reaction to women's friendships. There's an especially nice chapter on women's intimacy.

Real, Terrance. *I Don't Want to Talk About It* (Fireside, 1997).

This too is written for men, but we women are so eager to understand men better that this book is a real gem. There are particularly good chapters explaining men's winner/loser mentality, "hollow men" (those who are out of touch with their feelings), and the collateral damage that such hollowness causes.

Schwartzberg, Natalie, Kathy Berliner, and Demaris Jacob. *Single in a Married World: A Life Cycle Framework for Working with the Unmarried Adult* (W. W. Norton, 1995).

A first! Although written for mental health professionals, this book breaks new ground in providing guidelines for being an Always Single adult, from age 30 through old age. It puts into perspective the difficulty of being single in a society that really does value marriage more. It includes numerous examples of therapists sensitively working with Always Single women and men.

Secunda, Victoria. *Losing Your Parent, Finding Your Self* (Hyperion, 2000).

An easy read on a not-so-easy topic. If you've lost one or both parents, read this. If not, read this preventatively. It is a sensitive view of the impact of a parent's death on your identity and your relationship with your other parent, your siblings, your children, and your lovers.

Sheehy, Gail. *New Passages* (Random House, 1995).

Although not specifically addressing single women, this book describes the midlife decades for women and men—separately. There are the turbulent 30s, flourishing 40s, flaming 50s, and serene 60s. Plenty of examples help you find yourself and understand why you might have made some of the choices in your life, and how to think differently about those in the future.

Silverstein, Olga. *The Courage to Raise Good Men* (Viking, 1994).

Single mothers with sons, young or old, get thee to the bookstore, fast. Between the beginning story by the author of her early years in raising her son, to the last page by the author's then-45-year-old son, you will be rewarded. The author challenges the assumption that mothers need to separate from their sons.

Tannen, Deborah. *You Just Don't Understand* (Morrow, 1990).

This is a communication guidebook. The information is presented in a format that makes for easy discussions with men. Take any subsection at random and discuss it from each of your perspectives. Many of the arguments between men and women are really an outgrowth of not understanding each other's language.

Wolf, Naomi. *The Beauty Myth* (Vintage books, 1990).

Any time you find yourself worrying about your cellulite, reach out and read a chapter of this book—*any* chapter. You'll shudder at how you help the diet and cosmetic industries flourish. Wolf tackles the theme as it relates to work, violence, religion, and our culture in general.